The
Boston IVF
Handbook of Infertility

Acknowledgements

We would like to thank the other physicians and scientists at Boston IVF for their help and input into this project. We are also grateful to our wives and families for their patience and support of our endeavors.

The
Boston IVF
Handbook of
Infertility

A practical guide for practitioners
who care for infertile couples

Steven R. Bayer, MD
Michael M. Alper, MD and
Alan S. Penzias, MD

*Beth Israel Deaconess Medical Center and
Harvard Medical School, Boston, Massachusetts, USA*

The Parthenon Publishing Group
International Publishers in Medicine, Science & Technology

A CRC PRESS COMPANY
BOCA RATON   LONDON   NEW YORK   WASHINGTON, D.C.

About Boston IVF

Boston IVF was established in 1986 as one of the first freestanding IVF centers in the country. The unique practice model and commitment to the highest quality medical care for the infertile couple has resulted in continued growth and success within the organization. To this end, Boston IVF has established itself as the largest IVF center in the United States and has been responsible for the birth of more than 10 000 babies. Its affiliation with the Beth Israel Deaconess Medical Center and the Harvard Medical School has resulted in broad-based clinical and basic science research in the field of reproductive medicine. Boston IVF also has a strong commitment to education. There is active teaching of nurses, medical students, physicians in training and staff physicians. Through its commitment to quality patient care, medical research and education, Boston IVF is recognized as a world leader in infertility.

Library of Congress Cataloging-in-Publication Data
Data available on application

British Library Cataloguing in Publication Data
Bayer, Steven R.
    The Boston IVF handbook of infertility :
    a practical guide for practitioners who
    care for infertile couples
    1. Infertility
    I. Title. II. Alper, Michael M. III. Penzias,
    Alan S. IV. IVF Handbook of infertility
616.6'92

ISBN 1-84214-102-3

Published in the USA by
The Parthenon Publishing Group Inc.
345 Park Avenue South
10th Floor
New York, NY 10010, USA

Published in the UK and Europe by
The Parthenon Publishing Group Ltd.
23–25 Blades Court, Deodar Road
London SW15 2NU, UK

Copyright © 2002
The Parthenon Publishing Group

Typeset by AMA DataSet Ltd., Preston, UK
Printed and bound by Bookcraft (Bath) Ltd., Midsomer Norton, UK

Contents

Disclaimer

This handbook presents an understanding and a perspective of the current clinical and scientific advances in the field of reproductive medicine and infertility as of the date of its writing. The field of reproductive medicine and infertility is an emerging discipline and is subject to change. The information presented in this handbook should not be considered as dictating an exclusive course of treatment or procedure to be followed. Rather it is intended to be an educational aid to the physician on current information.

Foreword

The authors have written a needed book. Yes, another book on infertility is needed. They have incorporated up-to-date concepts and married them with a handbook (a 'how to' manual) in a very sophisticated fashion.

This is an exemplary contribution conveying a body of knowledge in regard to infertility. It is filled with important information, as well as clinical pearls gleaned from the literature as well as experience. Not only does it provide step-by-step techniques, it provides a philosophy of care. The breadth of the book is nothing short of amazing in that not only does it cover the pathogenesis and pathophysiology of infertility, but also looks at treatment both basic and sophisticated and ends with a practical compendium of consent forms, counseling and educational material. Even the bugaboo of practicing physicians, insurance and coding issues, are covered.

The book is extremely well illustrated with charts, graphs and tables that are very helpful to capture the ideas. In fact, one could just look at 'the pictures' and obtain a tremendous amount from this text. The work is well and efficiently referenced.

I feel comfortable in saying that anyone who would follow this book from preconception counseling to treatment, including *in vitro* fertilization, would serve their patients well and have a thorough grasp of the treatment of the infertile patient. The section on preconception counseling is extremely important since most of us glance over this important concept. The authors have included not only guidelines, but also internet resources on reproductive toxins.

Not only have they included consent forms, but they have also included a comprehensive history and physical form as well.

The paradigms for management are excellent as are the patient information sheets that are also included.

The book applies critical interpretation of some controversial areas, but is upbeat in most of its approach. The book is up to date including metformin treatment for polycystic ovary disease, a comprehensive approach to ectopic pregnancy including methotrexate and, of course, the latest protocols in regard to ART.

The book reminds me of the old time salesman who would step up on a corner, open up a case and in the case were his wares. Well, if this case is opened, this is all you need to know about infertility. It's all of infertility in a little black bag, 'Tell you what I'm going to do'.

Alan H. DeCherney, MD
Professor and Chair
Department of Obstetrics and Gynecology
UCLA School of Medicine
Los Angeles, CA, USA

1.
Overview of infertility

Over the past decade, there have been significant advances made in the field of reproductive medicine. The knowledge that has been gained has provided a better understanding of the pathophysiology of infertility and has resulted in the development of new and more effective therapies. With the introduction of these new therapies, there is a realization that infertility is not a simple medical problem. In addition to the medical component of infertility, there are psychological, genetic, legal, moral and social issues that must be considered. Therefore, a clinician who counsels and treats infertile couples must have the knowledge and understanding of the many issues encompassing infertility. This chapter serves to provide this essential knowledge.

DEFINITION

The traditional definition of infertility is the lack of conception after 1 year of unprotected intercourse. However, it must be realized that this time limit of 1 year is purely arbitrary. The monthly fecundity rate in the general population has been estimated to be between 15 and 20% and it can be expected that 86–94% of couples will have achieved a pregnancy after 12 months. Approximately 73–80% of pregnancies will be achieved in the first 6 months of trying. Taking into consideration the monthly fecundity rate in the general population, it is justified to perform an infertility evaluation and initiate treatment if a couple has failed to achieve a pregnancy after 6 months of trying. An evaluation may be indicated sooner if there is an obvious or known cause of the infertility (i.e. anovulation, blockage of the Fallopian tubes, etc.).

EPIDEMIOLOGY

Infertility is a prevalent problem in our society today. Over the past few years, the many issues surrounding infertility have become popular topics in the lay press. This has resulted in an increased awareness of infertility, but has also given the impression that we are amidst an epidemic of this problem. However, the

National Survey of Family Growth performed by the National Center for Health Statistics has provided insight into the prevalence of infertility in the United States[1]. This survey has been performed several times since 1960. When comparing the results from surveys performed over the past three decades, it can be concluded that the rate of infertility has not risen, but in fact has dropped slightly. In the most recent survey, performed in 1995, it was reported that 10.5% of women in the reproductive age group were infertile. In real numbers, this represents 6.1 million women in the United States. Despite the availability of medical treatment, only 21% of childless couples between the ages of 35 and 44 years ever sought infertility services.

IMPACT ON THE HEALTH-CARE SYSTEM

Many countries provide infertility services within their socialized medicine structure. However, insurance coverage for infertility treatment in the United States is left up to employers and insurance plans and is influenced by state insurance mandates. In essence, the majority of American women do not have insurance coverage for this medical problem. As of this writing, a total of 14 states have mandates that stipulate insurers to pay for infertility coverage but the degree of coverage varies from state to state. There is a stigma that must be overcome before we can hope for more extensive coverage. First, society does not view infertility as a medical problem and considers treatment to be elective, likened to plastic surgery. It is paradoxical that as a society there are no qualms about paying for the medical expenses for individuals who have been irresponsible and caused themselves harm with smoking or alcohol abuse. In contrast, for most infertile couples irresponsible behavior is not a cause of their plight. The solution is to define infertility as a medical problem and many states have done this to establish their state insurance mandates. In addition, in 1998 the Supreme Court ruled that reproduction is a major life activity under the American with Disabilities Act. The other misconception is that the costs of infertility treatment are a drain on the health-care system. This is in part fueled by the costly price tag of some of the treatments. For instance, the cost of an *in vitro* fertilization (IVF) cycle can range from $5000 to $15 000. The total expenditure on infertility services nationally is in the range of $2–3 billion per year. While this is a substantial amount of money, it is a fraction of the total money expended on health care in the United States, which in 1996 was estimated to be close to $1 trillion[2]. Further studies have concluded that if health-care plans offer comprehensive infertility services that the monthly family plan premium would go up by less than $2.00 per month.

FACTORS AFFECTING FERTILITY

As our knowledge has increased, there is a realization that there are many known and unknown factors that impact on fertility. Some of the more important factors that have been studied are discussed below.

Maternal age

One of the most important factors that influences a couple's fertility is the woman's age. A woman's fertility generally begins to decline after the age of 24 (Figure 1.1). When controlling for other factors, (i.e. decreased frequency of intercourse, age of the male partner, etc.) this age-related decrease in fertility is a real phenomenon. The most accepted explanation of decreased fertility is a decline in oocyte quality. It has been hypothesized that decreased oocyte quality increases the likelihood of meiotic and mitotic errors that could prevent normal fertilization and/or halt early embryonic development. In support of this hypothesis, studies performed on embryos resulting from *in vitro* fertilization have confirmed an increased incidence of aneuploidy in embryos obtained from older women[3]. The increased chance of chromosomal errors with advanced maternal age is further supported by the increased rate of spontaneous abortions and chromosomal anomalies in babies born to older women[4]. Another factor that is supported at least in animal studies is the presence of an age-related uterine dysfunction that could interfere with implantation. However, the pregnancies

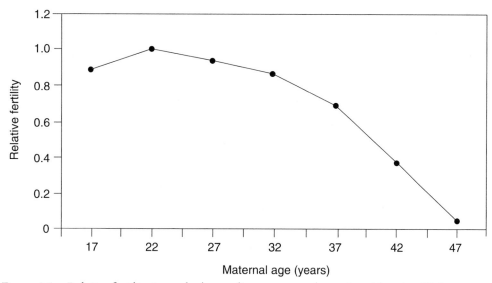

Figure 1.1 Relative fertility is graphed according to maternal age. An odds ratio of 1.0 was assigned to the 20–24 year age group that has the highest fertility rate. The data for this graph were modified from Coale AJ, Trussell TJ. *Popul Indes* 1974;40:185–256

that have been established in older women following egg donation treatment have weakened support for this hypothesis.

Paternal age

Like their female counterparts, males also experience a decrease in fertility associated with advancing age. However, males do retain their reproductive potential for a longer period of time and it is not uncommon for some men to retain their fertility into their sixth and seventh decades of life.

Frequency of intercourse

The frequency of intercourse is directly related to the chance of pregnancy. Maximal pregnancy rates are achieved when intercourse occurs on a daily basis around the time of ovulation. However, repeated ejaculations in males who have borderline sperm counts may cause a decrease in the semen volume and sperm concentration. In addition, some couples may find it difficult and stressful to have intercourse on a daily basis. Since sperm generally survive in the pre-ovulatory mucus for 3 or more days, we advise couples that intercourse every other day around the time of ovulation is sufficient.

Duration of attempting pregnancy

The average monthly fecundity rate in the general population is 15–20%. However, over time, the cumulative pregnancy rate continues to increase. Assuming a 15% monthly fecundity rate, the cumulative pregnancy rates at 4, 6 and 12 months are 48%, 62% and 86%, respectively. It can be concluded that the human reproductive system is inefficient and it is important that this fact be conveyed to our patients. This information is helpful and provides the proper perspective when couples are counseled about success rates following infertility treatment.

Other factors that impact on fertility

Previous contraception

The intrauterine device (IUD) increases the chances of pelvic inflammatory disease, which can lead to tubal damage. Women who have previously used an IUD are two times more likely to be infertile than women who have used other methods of contraception. The Dalcon Shield® IUD was the worse offender and increased the risk of infertility by six-fold[5]. Several years ago when the impact on fertility was realized, most of the IUDs were taken off the market. Over the past few years, IUDs have again become available and are considered an effective and safe contraceptive agent for parous women who are in a monogamous relationship. Used in this circumstance, the chance of a pelvic infection and subsequent infertility is significantly reduced.

One of the benefits of oral contraceptive use is a decreased incidence of a pelvic infection, which would help to preserve fertility. However, a previous study examined subsequent fertility in women who discontinued using various forms of contraception (oral contraceptives, barrier methods, intrauterine devices)[6]. Interestingly, the lowest monthly fecundity rate was noted in those women who discontinued oral contraceptives. The impairment in fertility was not related to the length of time the oral contraceptive was taken.

Occupational hazards

Toxins may be encountered in the work place that may affect reproductive health. It is well documented that there is a higher rate of spontaneous abortions in operating room personnel who are exposed to inhalation anesthetic agents. Exposure to other work-related chemicals (i.e. cadmium, mercury and dry cleaning chemicals) have also been reported to decrease fertility in women. The male is more susceptible to environmental toxins since spermatogenesis is an ongoing and dynamic process. DBCP (a pesticide), lead, ethylene glycol ethers, kepone (an insecticide), organic solvents and other chemicals have been shown to impact on male fertility.

Caffeine

There have been several reports linking a woman's caffeine intake to decreased fertility when controlling for other factors[7,8]. A dose-dependent relationship has been confirmed which suggests that any amount of caffeine consumption could be detrimental to fertility.

Smoking

The deleterious effects of smoking during pregnancy are well established. Several published studies have demonstrated that smoking is associated with decreased fertility[9,10]. Smoking can alter ovarian function in a number of ways[11]. First, the chemicals in smoke stimulate the hepatic metabolism of steroid hormones thereby reducing their levels in the blood stream. Second, *in vitro* studies have demonstrated that the chemicals in smoke alter the enzymes that are necessary for ovarian hormone production. Finally, women who smoke generally go through an earlier menopause by 1–2 years, suggesting that the chemicals in smoke may be directly toxic to the ovaries. It is not known whether this is due to a direct action on the ovaries or indirectly through an alteration of the blood flow to the ovary. Smoking affects male fertility, as well. Studies have confirmed that men who smoke have a reduction in all of the semen parameters including the concentration, motility and percentage of sperm with normal morphology.

Alcohol

The ill-effects of alcohol on pregnancy are well established. However, the influence of alcohol on fertility has not been well studied. In 1998, two separate studies were published that examined the impact of alcohol on the establishment of pregnancy[12,13]. Both studies arrived at the same conclusion that alcohol, in a dose-dependent fashion, reduced the chance of a conception in the study populations. There are no published data that suggest that moderate alcohol use affects male reproduction.

Stress

Infertility is associated with an intense psychological component, which can produce feelings of anxiety, guilt, inadequacy and overt depression. During the evaluation it is important that the clinician perform a psychological assessment on both the female and male partners to determine whether a referral to a mental health-care professional is indicated. There are no adequate studies indicating that stress actually causes infertility. Nevertheless, a previously published study reported on the benefits of relaxation techniques in reducing stress and potentially having a benefit on fertility[14]. Further research is needed to clarify the association of stress and fertility, and the benefits of any intervention.

OBJECTIVES OF THE INITIAL INTERVIEW

Since infertility is a problem that affects the couple, it is important that both partners are present for the initial interview and when decisions are made regarding treatment. Like any doctor–patient relationship it is important to establish good rapport but this is even more critical when one is caring for the infertile patient. Because of the psychological component that accompanies this diagnosis, patients with infertility require a much more demanding relationship than is required with other gynecological patients. The initial consultation is an important encounter and an adequate amount of time (30–60 min) should be spent with the couple. There are several objectives of the initial interview, which are described below.

Determine the necessity of an evaluation

Before an infertility work-up is begun it is important to make sure the couple meets the criteria for being infertile. One must determine whether the couple has had an adequate duration and exposure to potential pregnancy. Although the classic definition of infertility is the lack of pregnancy after 1 year of unprotected intercourse, we feel it is appropriate to initiate an evaluation after 6 months of infertility, or sooner if an obvious infertility factor is present or if the woman is older (> 39 years).

Educate the couple

It is important to educate the couple on normal reproductive function. Diagrams may be helpful in achieving this objective. A basic knowledge of the normal reproductive process helps the couple better understand the various causes of infertility, the rationale of the evaluation and the treatment that may be recommended.

Identify risk factors

Another objective of the initial interview is to identify risk factors that may explain the infertility. The identification of a risk factor would help to focus the evaluation. Irregularity of the menstrual cycles suggests an ovulatory problem. Previous use of an IUD puts a woman at risk of a pelvic infection that can result in tubal factor infertility. Complaints of dysmenorrhea or dyspareunia may suggest the presence of endometriosis. Previous conization or cryosurgery of the cervix increases the chance of a cervical factor.

Preconceptional care

An important part of the initial consultation is a discussion on preconceptional care. This involves a review of medical, environmental, nutritional, social and genetic issues that may complicate the outcome of a pregnancy. In some cases, the particular issue of concern must be investigated before proceeding with any treatment. An in-depth discussion of preconceptional care appears in Chapter 2 of this handbook.

Treatment plan

At the end of the consultation, a plan for evaluation should be discussed with the couple. The couple should have a good understanding about the scope of the evaluation and the rationale for the tests that have been selected. Written material should be given to the couple describing the tests that will be performed. Finally, the couple should be given an estimate of the length of time to complete the evaluation and when to schedule a follow-up appointment to discuss the results and begin discussions about treatment.

CAUSES OF INFERTILITY

The causes of infertility can be varied and in many cases a combination of factors is identified. An objective of the infertility evaluation is to identify specific cause(s) of the infertility, which will allow the clinician to administer the appropriate treatment (Figure 1.2). In years past, there was much emphasis placed on the infertility evaluation, which was elaborate and could take a significant amount of time to complete. The standard infertility evaluation involved the performance of several tests, including the semen analysis, hystero-salpingogram, postcoital test, endometrial biopsy and a laparoscopy. During the course of the evaluation it was not uncommon that the postcoital test and endometrial biopsy were repeated multiple times; however, published studies have confirmed that these tests are unreliable and do not differentiate between fertile and infertile populations. In the past, it was also common practice to perform a laparoscopy before any therapy was started. However, we now realize that, in many cases, the findings at the time of the laparoscopy do not change the course of recommended treatment. To this end, the infertility evaluation has been redefined and is now more efficient, informative and cost-effective (Table 1.1). A discussion of the various causes of infertility and the current infertility evaluation is presented. The reader is also referred to Chapter 4 where clinical algorithms are presented.

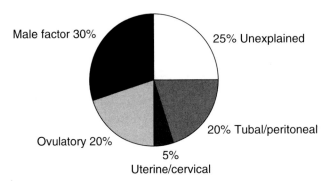

Figure 1.2 Causes of infertility

Table 1.1   Past and present tests used for evaluation of infertility

Past	Present
Semen analysis	semen analysis
Endometrial biopsy	cycle day 3 FSH/estradiol
Hysterosalpingogram	hysterosalpingogram
Postcoital test	preconceptional care
Laparoscopy	laparoscopy (optional)

Ovarian function

One of the first steps in the infertility evaluation is to assess ovarian function. Significant information can be obtained from the menstrual history including the age at menarche, frequency of menstrual cycles in the present and past, and the duration of menstrual flow. Important aspects of ovarian function related to fertility are discussed below.

Determination of whether ovulation is occurring

If a woman is having regular menstrual cycles that are 23–39 days in length then she is ovulating. This is further supported if the bleeding is preceded by premenstrual symptoms (i.e. water weight gain, breast tenderness and mood changes). If there is any doubt about a woman's ovulatory status then a simple inexpensive test is to have her keep a daily record of her temperature. The progesterone that is secreted by the corpus luteum during the luteal phase acts on the temperature-regulating center in the hypothalamus causing an increase in the basal temperature from 0.5–1.0°F. In the past, women have been instructed to take their temperature upon wakening; however, the temperature can be taken at other times of the day as long as it is done on a consistent basis. There will be an occasional patient who is not compliant in keeping a basal body temperature chart or whose temperature chart cannot be interpreted. In these instances, a serum progesterone determination may be helpful and a level greater than 3 ng/ml confirms that ovulation has occurred. The use of ovulation predictor kits have become quite popular over the past several years. If a woman notes a positive test using the ovulation predictor kit this is yet another confirmatory test that ovulation is taking place.

Luteal phase deficiency

In the past, there was a belief that luteal phase deficiency was a cause of infertility and recurrent miscarriages. It was theorized that some women may be ovulating and having regular menstrual cycles but the progesterone secreted during the luteal phase is insufficient to mature the endometrium for implantation or unable to support a pregnancy. There were two approaches to the evaluation of the adequacy of the luteal phase. The first was measuring a mid-luteal phase progesterone level. If the level was below 10 ng/ml then this was suggestive of a progesterone deficiency. The major difficulty with using progesterone levels in this fashion is that progesterone is secreted in pulses every 2–3 hours, which will interfere with the interpretation of a single level. The more popular technique to assess the adequacy of the luteal phase was an endometrial biopsy performed late in the luteal phase. It was thought that the endometrial biopsy represented a bioassay of all of the progesterone that was secreted during the luteal phase. Progesterone secreted in the luteal phase causes day-by-day changes in the endometrium that can be appreciated histologically. A luteal phase deficiency was established if there was at least a 3-day lag between the histological date of the endometrial biopsy and the chronological date of the menstrual cycle (established retrospectively with the knowledge of the onset of the next menses and assuming a 14-day luteal phase). From a theoretical standpoint this makes good sense, but there are problems with the endometrial biopsy for assessment of the luteal phase, including:

(1) Uncertainty when the menstrual period begins which would interfere with the establishment of the chronological day;

(2) Interobserver variation in the pathological interpretation of the biopsy;

(3) The false premise that the luteal phase is 14 days in length, which can actually range between 13 and 16 days;

(4) 20% of *fertile* women will have an out-of-phase endometrial biopsy.

The data published to date raise questions about the diagnosis of luteal phase deficiency[15–17]. Taking this into consideration, plus the unreliability of the testing and the lack of proof of treatment efficacy, we do not feel that assessment of the luteal phase should be a part of the infertility evaluation.

Assessment of ovarian reserve

During a woman's lifetime, the maximum number of oocytes is present *in utero* at 20 weeks of gestation. From then on, there is a gradual and progressive decrease in the ovarian reserve of oocytes. Ultimately, there is total depletion of the oocytes and menopause results. It must be realized that menopause is not an abrupt process but represents an end-point to a transitional process that spans

Table 1.2 Interpretation of cycle day 3 hormone levels

Follicle stimulating hormone level* (mIU/ml)	Estradiol level† (pg/ml)	Ovarian reserve
> 10	< 70	↓
> 10	> 70	↓
2–10	> 70	↓
2–10	<70	normal

* Normal FSH level 2–10 mIU/ml; †normal estradiol level < 70 pg/ml

several years. One of the first changes that a woman can notice as she approaches menopause is a gradual shortening of the menstrual cycle. In addition, early follicular phase follicle stimulating hormone (FSH) and estradiol levels also can identify women who are starting to approach the menopausal transition. An elevated FSH (> 10 mIU/ml) or estradiol (> 70 pg/ml) measurement during the early follicular phase (cycle days 2–4) suggests the presence of reduced ovarian reserve (Table 1.2).

The clomiphene citrate challenge test is a dynamic test used to examine ovarian reserve. Clomiphene citrate is a weak estrogen agonist that binds to estrogen receptors in the hypothalamus which results in the release of FSH and luteinizing hormone (LH) from pituitary gonadotrophs. The test involves the following:

Clomiphene citrate challenge test
1. Cycle day 3 – FSH + estradiol levels
2. Clomiphene citrate 100 mg cycle days 5–9
3. Cycle day 10 – FSH level

Interpretation: If any of the FSH levels are > 10 mIU/ml or the estradiol is > 70 pg/ml the test is considered abnormal and confirms reduced ovarian reserve.

If any of the FSH levels are greater than 10 mIU/ml or the day-3 estradiol is greater than 70 pg/ml, it can be concluded that reduced ovarian reserve is present. The clomiphene citrate challenge test can be more informative since 75% of women with reduced ovarian reserve have a normal cycle day 3 hormone assessment.

Reduced ovarian reserve is associated with a reduced chance of pregnancy and a higher chance of miscarriage[18]. This information helps the clinician in counseling the couple on treatment options. However, there are limitations in the correlation between the FSH levels and fertility. We have observed that some women have slightly elevated FSH levels but normal fertility. We have also confirmed that some women have fluctuations in the FSH levels from cycle to cycle and over time.

Assessment of ovarian reserve should be performed routinely and should include a FSH and estradiol level measured between cycle days 2 and 4. Any woman who has evidence of reduced ovarian reserve should be referred for counseling and offered aggressive treatment.

Evaluation of the woman with ovulatory dysfunction

Ovulatory dysfunction is present in a woman who has menstrual cycles that are out of the normal range (25–35 days). The initial work-up should include measurement of thyroid stimulating hormone (TSH), prolactin, and cycle day 3 FSH and estradiol levels. Prolactin levels fluctuate throughout the day reaching a nadir in the morning and tend to be higher in the luteal phase. Therefore, it is important that the prolactin determination be performed on a morning follicular phase blood sample. If the woman has symptoms of hyperandrogenism, then additional testing is indicated. This should include a determination of testosterone, dehydroepiandrosterone sulfate (DHEAS) and 17-hydroxy-progesterone (17-OHP) levels. The 17-OHP determination should also be performed on a morning follicular phase blood sample. There is new evidence that insulin resistance can be the cause of chronic anovulation. Therefore, in addition to the androgen studies, a fasting glucose and insulin level should be assessed. If the glucose to insulin ratio is less than 4.5, then insulin resistance should be suspected[19]. Those women with insulin resistance should undergo screening for diabetes mellitus with a fasting plasma glucose determination.

The clinical presentation and the laboratory studies will help to determine the cause of the ovulatory dysfunction, which can be varied and secondary to hypothalamic dysfunction (reduced weight), chronic anovulation (polycystic ovarian disease) and impending ovarian failure. For an overview of the work-up of ovulatory dysfunction, refer to clinical algorithms in Chapter 4.

Cervical factor infertility

The cervix plays an important role in reproductive physiology. It provides the passageway for sperm allowing them access into the uterine cavity and ultimately the Fallopian tubes. The ability of the sperm to gain access to the upper tract is influenced by the cervical mucus that is present in the cervical canal. The estradiol that is produced by the pre-ovulatory follicle increases the quantity and consistency of mucus produced by the endocervical glands. Estradiol increases the water content of the mucus that reaches a peak of

95–98% at mid-cycle. In the days that precede ovulation, a thin, watery mucus spills out of the cervical canal and covers the portio of the cervix and upper vagina. Some women notice this change in the cervical mucus, whereas, others do not. If intercourse occurs during this time period the sperm are able to penetrate the mucus and survive for up to 3 days or more. In contrast, during the early follicular phase when the estradiol levels are low or in the luteal phase when any estrogenic affect is counteracted by progesterone, the cervical mucus is thick and tenacious. If intercourse occurs at these times the sperm are unable to penetrate this poor quality mucus and the sperm die in the vagina within a few hours because of its acidic environment.

Impaired sperm penetration of the cervical mucus following intercourse can prevent the establishment of pregnancy. The etiology of this condition is varied and can be secondary to faulty coital technique, inadequate cervical mucus production or poor quality sperm. Less than 5% of infertile couples will have a cervical factor as the cause of their infertility (excluding couples with a contributory male factor). A previous history of conization of the cervix, or ablative surgery to the cervix can put the woman at risk for a cervical factor. It is also important to ask couples about the use of lubricants during intercourse. Lubricants such as K-Y® jelly and Surgilube® can impair sperm motility. An alternative is vegetable oil, which does not impair sperm function.

The postcoital test

The postcoital test is the diagnostic test that has been used to assess the functional capacity of the cervix as it relates to fertility. The postcoital test is an evaluation of the quality of the cervical mucus and a determination of the number of sperm that have penetrated the mucus. There has been controversy about the test in part because it has never been standardized. Further, published data have confirmed that the postcoital test is unreliable and does not differentiate between fertile and infertile couples[20].

Taking into consideration the published data, it is our opinion that the postcoital test should not be part of the routine evaluation. However, an assessment of the cervical mucus during the pre-ovulatory period may be indicated in the woman who has had a destructive procedure performed on the cervix, which may compromise cervical mucus production.

Male factor infertility

Male factor infertility is common and is identified in approximately 30% of infertile couples. At the initial consultation, it is important that an in-depth medical history is obtained from the male partner. Previous surgery for repair of an inguinal hernia could have resulted in inadvertent injury to the vas deferens, which courses through the inguinal canal. A history of cryptorchidism can be associated with altered testicular function. Chronic illnesses (i.e. chronic renal disease, thyroid dysfunction, diabetes mellitus and malnourished states) can also impair normal spermatogenesis. A neuropathy can complicate diabetes and can result in the development of impotence or retrograde ejaculation.

A medication history is also important. Sulfasalizine can be prescribed for ulcerative colitis and cause a decrease in sperm concentration and motility, which will resolve after the medication is discontinued. The antimitotic activity of colchicine, a medication prescribed for gout, can also decrease sperm production. Some medications that are used to treat hypertension and mood disorders have sympathetic or parasympathetic actions that can interfere with erectile function and/or ejaculation. Male body builders should be questioned about the use of anabolic steroids and other oral hormonal agents that can result in significant oligospermia and in some cases azoospermia. Other medications that can impact on male reproduction include the following: cimetidine, spironolactone, isoniazid, calcium channel blockers and chemotherapeutic drugs. Recreational drugs such as alcohol, tobacco and marijuana if taken in excess can also be detrimental. Spermatogenesis is a temperature-sensitive process and the scrotal temperature is generally 2–3°F lower than core body temperature. Hot tubs, saunas or a febrile illness can increase the temperature of the testes and can impair sperm production. Finally, the male should be questioned regarding chemical exposures at the workplace. Exposure to insecticides, pesticides, lead and organic solvents, among others, have been shown to impact on male fertility.

The semen analysis has been the standard test for the evaluation of the male partner. The male partner is instructed to abstain from ejaculation for 2 days prior to performance of the test. The specimen is produced by masturbation. Depending on the laboratory facility the specimen can be produced on site. If the couple lives within 45 minutes of the laboratory then the sample can be produced at home and then transported to the laboratory for the analysis. During transport, it is important that the sample is kept at body temperature. The normal parameters of the semen analysis are shown in Table 1.3.

An important assessment of the semen analysis is a determination of the percentage of sperm with normal morphology (Figure 1.3). The World Health Organization (WHO) classification system has been used to evaluate sperm morphology. It is considered normal if ≥ 40% of the sperm have normal morphology. Presently, the Tygerberg and Krüger classification systems are widely used and are more critical assessments of sperm morphology. By these

Table 1.3 Normal parameters of semen analysis

Volume	2–5 cc
Sperm count	> 20 million sperm/cc
Motility	> 50%
Morphology	> 4% normal forms (by Krüger classification)
	> 40% normal forms (by World Health Organization criteria)
Liquefaction time	15–30 min

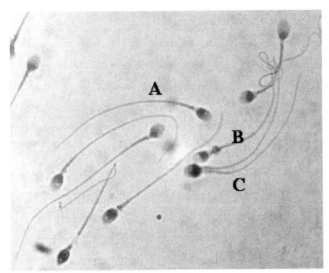

Figure 1.3 A standard part of the semen analysis is an assessment of the morphology or shape of the sperm. Note: a spermatozoon with normal morphology (A), and spermatozoa with abnormal morphology including one with a mid-piece defect (B) and one with two tails (C)

classifications, it is considered normal if > 4% of the sperm have normal morphology. Since a semen analysis is a specialized test, it is important to select an experienced laboratory to perform the test. The reliability of the interpretation of a semen sample will be proportional to the number of specimens that are handled by any particular laboratory.

If the semen analysis is normal then no further work-up of the male partner is indicated. If the semen analysis is abnormal then a repeat sample should be obtained 3–4 weeks later. There is day-to-day variability of the semen parameters. Further, an abnormal semen analysis might be explained by a stressful event (i.e. febrile illness) that occurred 2–3 months prior to the time of the initial semen analysis. This is the amount of time it takes for mature sperm to develop.

In the past, it was routine to refer the male partner to a urologist for an examination of the genitals and to determine whether a varicocele was present. A varicocele is a dilated scrotal vein, which can be identified in up to 25% of infertile males but can also be present in 10–15% of normal fertile males. There are several theories that have been proposed to explain the association between the varicocele and male infertility. The most accepted theory is that the dilated testicular vein raises the temperature of the testes, which alters sperm production. However, controversy continues about the association of a varicocele and infertility, and the benefits of surgical correction. The reported pregnancy rates following surgical ligation of a varicocele are between 30 and 50%. However, a meta-analysis of pertinent studies failed to demonstrate any improvement in male fertility following a varicocele ligation[21].

Laboratory studies (FSH, LH, testosterone, and prolactin) may help to rule out an endocrinopathy, which could explain significantly impaired spermatogenesis. If the gonadotropins (FSH, LH) are depressed or undetectable, this may suggest the presence of either Kallman's syndrome or hypothalamic dysfunction, which can be corrected with FSH and human chorionic gonadotropin (hCG), or gonadotropin releasing hormone (GnRH) treatment. An elevated FSH level suggests the presence of testicular failure that is usually unexplained but may be secondary to Kleinfelter's syndrome (47,XXY), Sertoli-only-cell syndrome, previous mumps orchitis or prior cancer treatment. Hyperprolactinemia is uncommon in the male but can be associated with impotence. In the male with azoospermia and normal gonadotropins, one must consider either the presence of an obstructed outflow tract or congenital absence of the vas deferens as the cause. Often the diagnosis can be made on physical examination but a testicular biopsy with a vasogram may be helpful. While a physical examination and laboratory evaluation are helpful to evaluate the male with abnormal semen parameters, the majority of cases remain unexplained.

It is important to realize that the semen analysis is a quantitative assessment of the semen sample. Unfortunately, we do not have a test that provides a qualitative assessment of sperm function short of *in vitro* fertilization or pregnancy itself. Several years ago the hamster penetration assay was touted as a qualitative test of sperm function but numerous studies have disproved its reliability and we do not feel that it has any use in the evaluation of the male infertility.

Tubal factor infertility

Tubal factor infertility is present in approximately 20% of infertile women. Risk factors include a previous ectopic pregnancy, ruptured appendix, previous use of an IUD or a past history of pelvic inflammatory disease. Even so, the majority of women who are found to have a tubal factor do not have any risk factor. These cases are most likely the result of an asymptomatic pelvic infection.

The hysterosalpingogram (HSG) is the standard test to assess tubal patency (Figures 1.4 and 1.5). This test is performed early in the follicular phase after the cessation of menstrual flow. It is safer to use a water-based medium for the examination. Absolute contraindications for performing the test are suspicion of pregnancy and active pelvic infection. A complication following a HSG is an infection, which has an incidence of 1–3%[22]. For this reason, prophylactic antibiotics (i.e. metronidazole, doxycycline) should be considered for women who have a history of a sexually transmitted disease or a pelvic infection or who are diagnosed with a hydrosalpinx at the time of the HSG. If the woman has a known iodine allergy or has had any allergic reaction to fish or shellfish, the test should be reconsidered. If the allergy is mild, the test can be performed with a

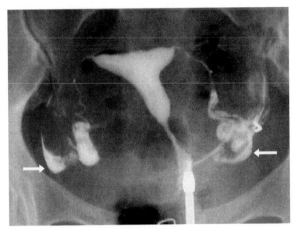

Figure 1.4   Normal hysterosalpingogram (HSG). This HSG demonstrates a uterine cavity that has a normal shape and there are no filling defects noted within the cavity. Both Fallopian tubes have filled and the arrows point to dye that has exited the ends of both tubes into the abdominal cavity

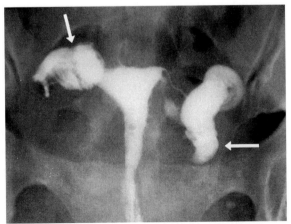

Figure 1.5   Distal tubal obstruction. In this X-ray both Fallopian tubes are filled but their distal ends are dilated and no dye is seen escaping into the abdominal cavity. The ends of the tubes are indicated by the arrows. This finding is most likely the result of a pelvic infection

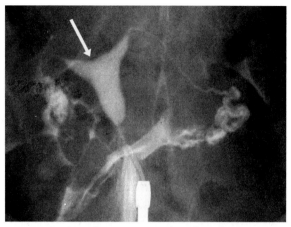

Figure 1.6 Arcuate uterus. In this otherwise normal study a depression can be seen indenting the superior aspect of the uterine cavity (see arrow). This is compatible with an arcuate uterus and is considered a normal variant. No additional work-up is indicated. For comparison, a normal uterine cavity can be seen in Figures 1.4 and 1.5

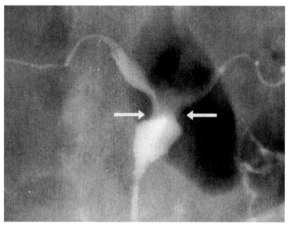

Figure 1.7 A diethylstilbestrol (DES) uterus. The shape of this uterine cavity is compatible with previous DES exposure that causes impingement of the lateral walls as indicated by the arrows. The prominent uterine horns create a bicornuate shape, as well. Overall the uterine cavity has a 'T-shape' which is classic for previous DES exposure

contrast medium that contains non-ionic iodine, which reduces the chance of an allergic reaction. If the woman has a more significant iodine allergy, the clinician should consult with the radiologist before performing the test.

In addition to assessing tubal patency, the HSG allows examination of the uterine cavity (Figures 1.6–1.11). To examine the uterine cavity adequately if a balloon catheter is used, the balloon should be deflated at the end of the examination while the contrast medium is injected. We routinely attach a tenaculum to the anterior cervix for traction and inject the dye through a cannula with a plastic cone-shaped tip that is abutted against the external cervical os. Retraction of the tenaculum caudad straightens out the uterus and

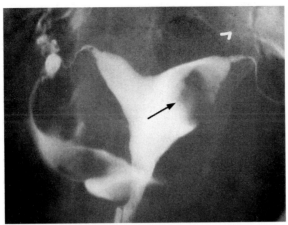

Figure 1.8 Submucosal fibroid. This hysterosalpingogram demonstrates a large filling defect in the left uterine horn, which was later found to be a submucosal fibroid. Also note the depression in the superior aspect of the cavity which is an arcuate deformity

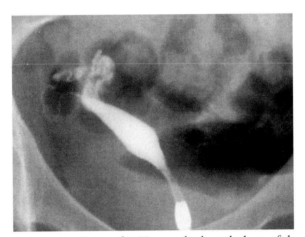

Figure 1.9 Unicornuate uterus. During this X-ray only the right horn of the uterine cavity filled. This is compatible with a unicornuate uterus. A unicornuate uterus increases the risk of premature labor and malpresentations. It can be accompanied by renal abnormalities

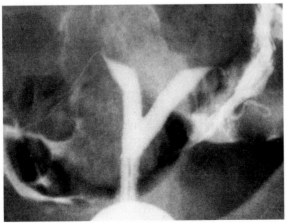

Figure 1.10 Uterine septum. This X-ray demonstrates a division in the uterine cavity, which was confirmed to be a uterine septum

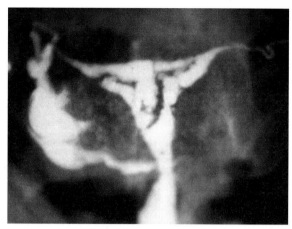

Figure 1.11 Asherman's syndrome. This patient presented with infertility following a dilatation and curettage for a missed abortion. Note the dark irregular areas in the cavity, which can be explained by intrauterine adhesions

allows a better examination of the cavity. If the dye is injected slowly and if a non-steroidal anti-inflammatory drug is given prior to the procedure, the HSG can be performed with minimal discomfort or even painlessly contrary to popular belief.

Besides being a diagnostic tool, the HSG has been shown to be of therapeutic benefit as well. Approximately 30% of patients who have a normal HSG will conceive over the following 6 months[23]. Initially, this was thought to be only a characteristic of the oil-based contrast medium. A prospective randomized study demonstrated comparable pregnancy rates over a 6-month period in patients who had tubal patency confirmed either using a water- or an oil-based contrast medium[23]. In an effort to explain the therapeutic benefit of the HSG, some have suggested that the injection of dye may dislodge intratubal mucus plugs, stimulate the tubal cilia or break up intratubal adhesions.

When is a laparoscopy indicated?

A laparoscopy is the most invasive of the infertility tests and, for this reason, is generally performed after the completion of the work-up. In the past, it was considered a routine part of the infertility evaluation, but presently we counsel our patients on the risks and benefits of the procedure and perform it on an individual basis. There are some women who choose to have a laparoscopy during the initial part of the evaluation while others choose never to have the surgery performed and proceed with treatment. A laparoscopy may be more seriously considered for the patient who has a history of a pelvic infection, signs or symptoms compatible with endometriosis, or abnormal findings on the HSG. It is important that the findings at the time of surgery are clearly documented not only with an accurate operative note, but drawings, pictures and video recordings are also helpful. At the time of the laparoscopy, the surgeon must have the necessary tools available to treat any conditions that are encountered. If endometriosis is identified the patient should be properly staged. Staging sheets can be obtained by contacting the American Society of Reproductive Medicine in Birmingham, Alabama (see Chapter 12) or obtaining a copy of the article entitled 'Revised American Society for Reproductive Medicine classification of endometriosis' (*Fertil Steril* 1997;67:817–21). In some cases, the performance of a hysteroscopy may also be warranted.

If bilateral distal tubal obstruction is identified on the HSG, a laparoscopy is not always necessary and the patient can go directly to *in vitro* fertilization treatment.

Uterine factor infertility

Dysfunction in the uterus can prevent the establishment of a pregnancy. Further evaluation of the uterine cavity should be considered for any woman who has abnormal bleeding, an abnormal cavity noted on the HSG or a history of repeated miscarriages. Uterine fibroids are a common finding and occur in approximately 15–20% of women over the age of 35. In the majority of cases, the fibroids do not produce symptoms or impact on fertility. Fibroids can be located and attached to the outside of the uterus (subserosal), in the uterine wall (intramural) and in the cavity (submucosal). It is the submucosal fibroids that can have the greatest impact on fertility.

The HSG provides a good examination of the cavity but the examination can be somewhat limited. When the clinician is suspicious of an abnormality in the cavity then further testing may be indicated with a hysteroscopy or a sonohysterogram (SHG). We have found the SHG to be an excellent test to evaluate the cavity. This is a test that can be performed in the office if the clinician has access to a vaginal ultrasound. To perform the test a small catheter is inserted into the cavity and a syringe filled with saline is attached. Then the vaginal ultrasound is inserted. After the uterus is identified saline is injected into the cavity. A normal cavity has sharp borders (Figure 1.12). If any structure is seen in the cavity then it is considered abnormal and could represent a polyp or fibroid (Figure 1.13). In this circumstance, a hysteroscopic examination would be indicated.

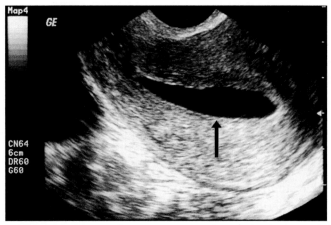

Figure 1.12 Sonohysterogram (normal cavity). This is a longitudinal image of the uterus taken at the time of a sonohysterogram. The black area (arrow) is the image of the saline that has been injected into the uterine cavity. Note that the borders of the uterine cavity are sharp and no masses are noted to be entering into the cavity. This study confirms a normal uterine cavity

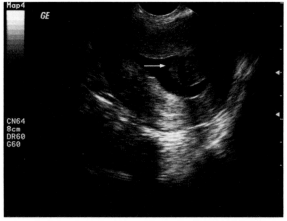

Figure 1.13 Sonohysterogram (abnormal cavity). In this image the injected fluid in the cavity (appearing black) outlines an intracavitary mass, which was later confirmed to be a uterine fibroid

CONCLUSIONS

The causes of infertility can be varied and the infertility evaluation will provide a better understanding of the potential causes. Up to 25% of couples will have a combination of factors and, therefore, it is important that a complete evaluation is performed and the evaluation is not halted after an abnormal test is encountered. After the evaluation is completed then the couple should be seen in consultation to discuss the results and formulate a treatment plan.

Recommended reading

- Adamson D, Chang RJ, DeCherney AH, *et al.* A model for initial care of the infertile couple. *J Reprod Med* 2001;46(Suppl 4):409–26
- Yen SSC, Jaffe RB, Barbieri RL. *Reproductive Endocrinology*. Philadelphia: W.B. Saunders Company, 1999
- Speroff L, Glass RH, Kase NG. *Clinical Gynecologic Endocrinology and Infertility*. Baltimore: Williams & Wilkins, 1999
- American Society for Reproductive Medicine. *Optimal Evaluation of the Infertile Female. A Practical Committee Report; A Committee Opinion.* Birmingham, ALA: American Society for Reproductive Medicine, 2000

2.

Preconceptional care

INTRODUCTION

The goal of treatment of the infertile couple goes beyond just simply the establishment of a pregnancy, but should be the establishment of a pregnancy that is uncomplicated and results in the delivery of a healthy baby. In some cases, the woman has a medical condition, is taking a medication, has a genetic risk or is exposed to an environmental toxin that during pregnancy could jeopardize her health and/or the health of her unborn child. To this end, an important aspect of treating infertile couples (or any couple contemplating a pregnancy) is preconceptional care, which is an assessment of medical, social, genetic, environmental and occupational factors that can impact on fertility and the health of a pregnancy (Figure 2.1). In some cases, the issue of concern must be investigated before any treatment is begun. In this chapter, a comprehensive summary and framework for preconceptional care is presented.

LIFESTYLE HABITS

A social history with an assessment of lifestyle habits is an important part of the medical history that should be obtained from the male and female partners. The use of tobacco, alcohol and recreational drugs should be ascertained and the couples appropriately counseled. These habits may not only be harmful during pregnancy but could also impair conception.

Smoking

Smoking is one of the major public health-care issues that continues to challenge the medical community today. Approximately 30% of women in the reproductive age group smoke. The impact of smoking on general health is well known. There are substantial data to support that smoking compromises reproductive health and, therefore can be considered a reproductive toxin[11]. Women who smoke are at greater risk of having infertility, a spontaneous abortion and a tubal pregnancy. During pregnancy maternal smoking increases the chances of

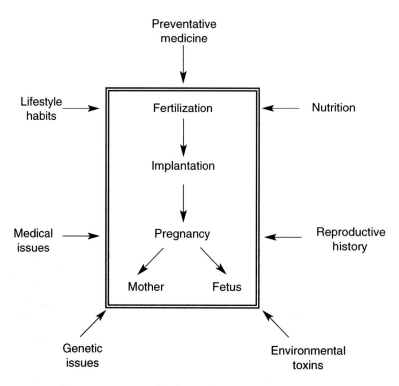

Figure 2.1 Factors that can impact on fertility and pregnancy

abruptio placenta, premature rupture of the membranes and impaired fetal growth. Maternal smoking during pregnancy also increases the chance of the sudden infant death syndrome (SIDS). It is clear that any woman who smokes and is contemplating a pregnancy should be strongly encouraged to stop. Smoking is a strong addiction and a referral for active intervention is indicated.

Alcohol

Alcohol use during pregnancy increases the risk of several complications and the complication of most concern is fetal alcohol syndrome, which is associated with altered fetal growth, dysmorphic features and mental retardation. The risk of fetal alcohol syndrome is related to the degree of alcohol intake but unfortunately no level of alcohol intake is considered safe. In addition, alcohol can impair fertility. Previous studies have demonstrated that any degree of alcohol intake by the woman can decrease the chances of conception[12,13]. Therefore, we recommend that if a woman is trying to achieve a pregnancy that she should either eliminate alcohol from her diet or limit its use to the first week of the menstrual cycle. Heavy alcohol intake may suggest an addiction and a history of other drug use should be ascertained. In some cases, a referral for counseling may be indicated before the couple attempts a pregnancy.

Recreational drug use

The use of recreational drugs is absolutely contraindicated while a couple is attempting to conceive and during pregnancy. Males who use marijuana on a regular basis have lower serum testosterone levels and decreased sperm counts. Other drugs used by the mother, such as cocaine and heroine, may lead to severe withdrawal reactions in the baby after it is born. Further, the use of intravenous drugs increases the risk of human immunodeficiency virus (HIV) and hepatitis infections. If there is concern over previous or ongoing drug use, a referral for counseling may be indicated.

NUTRITION

There is no doubt that our general health is influenced by what we eat, how much we eat and how much energy we expend with activity and exercise. In addition, nutrition impacts on reproductive health, as well, and can influence the establishment and maintenance of a pregnancy. As a general recommendation, women should be encouraged to maintain a balanced diet of fruits, vegetables, breads, meats and dairy products. Foods with a high content of fats and oils should be used at a minimum (Figure 2.2). In addition to a well-balanced diet, caloric intake should be limited to maintain a normal body weight. However, there are increased caloric demands and weight gain that are

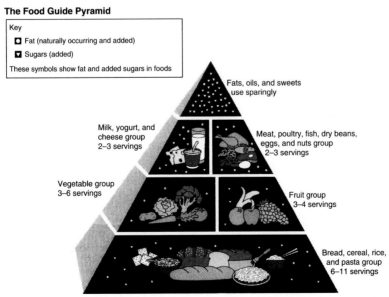

Figure 2.2 Food guide pyramid. Reproduced from US Department of Agriculture and the US Department of Health and Human Services, 1996

expected during pregnancy. Other important aspects of nutrition and diet are discussed below.

Body weight

Extremes of body weight can be associated with altered ovarian function. It is well established that a threshold body weight and fat content are necessary to maintain normal ovarian function. If the body weight is reduced below the 10th percentile for a particular height (body mass index (BMI) < 18; see below for calculation of BMI) or the body fat content is reduced to less than 22%, then altered menstrual function and ovulatory dysfunction can develop[24]. This explains the high incidence of amenorrhea in some female athletes (e.g. marathon runners, ballet dancers) and women who diet excessively. Alternatively, increased body weight can also be associated with ovulatory dysfunction. A major concern about increased body weight is the increased incidence of complications that may occur during pregnancy including diabetes, hypertension and thromboembolism. Women who are overweight tend to have larger babies, which increases the chance of shoulder dystocia and the need for a Cesarean section. A Cesarean section that is performed on a woman who is overweight is associated with a higher incidence of anesthetic and surgical complications. Obesity is responsible for 18% of maternal mortalities and 80% of anesthesia-related mortalities[25].

Assessing the body habitus

The body mass index (BMI) or the Quetelet's index is a determination of whether an individual's weight is appropriate. It is a calculation that takes into account the weight and height (weight (kg)/height (m^2)). A reference table to calculate the BMI is provided. An easy way to calculate the BMI is as follows: multiply the weight in pounds by 704 then divide by height (in inches) squared.

> *Example*   A woman is 5′ (60″) tall and weighs 207 lbs. Her BMI would be calculated as follows:
>
> BMI = $207 \times 704/60^2 = 40.5$

The BMI is a quantitative measure that helps to put into perspective the individual's weight. A woman is considered *normal* if the BMI is 18.5–24.9, *overweight* if the BMI is 25–29.9, *obese* if the BMI is 30–39.9 and *extremely obese* if the BMI is 40 or higher[26].

BODY MASS INDEX

	Normal						Overweight					Obesity										Extreme obesity					
	19	20	21	22	23	24	25	26	27	28	29	30	31	32	33	34	35	36	37	38	39	40	41	42	43	44	45
4'10"	91	96	100	105	110	115	119	124	129	134	138	143	148	153	158	162	167	172	177	181	186	191	196	201	205	210	215
4'11"	94	99	104	109	114	119	124	128	133	138	143	148	153	158	163	168	173	178	183	188	193	196	203	208	212	215	222
5'0"	97	102	107	112	118	123	128	133	138	143	148	153	158	163	169	173	179	184	189	194	199	204	209	215	220	225	230
5'1"	100	106	111	116	122	127	132	137	143	148	153	158	164	169	174	180	185	190	195	201	206	211	217	222	227	232	238
5'2"	104	10	115	120	126	131	136	142	147	153	158	164	169	174	180	185	191	196	202	207	213	218	224	229	235	240	246
5'3"	107	113	118	124	130	135	141	146	152	158	163	169	175	180	185	192	197	203	208	214	220	225	231	237	242	248	254
5'4"	110	116	122	128	134	140	145	151	157	163	169	174	180	186	192	197	204	209	215	221	227	232	238	244	250	256	262
5'5"	114	120	126	132	138	144	150	156	162	168	14	180	186	192	198	204	210	216	222	228	234	240	246	252	258	264	270
5'6"	118	124	130	136	142	148	155	161	167	173	179	186	192	198	204	210	216	223	229	235	241	247	253	260	266	272	278
5'7"	121	127	134	140	146	153	159	166	172	178	185	191	198	204	211	217	223	230	236	242	249	255	261	268	274	280	287
5'8"	125	131	138	144	151	158	164	171	177	184	190	197	203	210	216	223	230	236	243	249	256	262	269	276	282	289	295
5'9"	128	135	142	149	155	162	169	176	182	189	196	203	209	216	223	230	236	243	250	257	263	270	277	284	291	297	304
5'10"	132	139	146	153	160	167	174	181	188	195	202	209	216	222	229	236	243	250	257	264	271	278	285	292	299	306	313
5'11"	136	143	150	157	165	172	179	186	193	200	208	215	222	229	236	243	250	257	265	272	279	286	293	301	308	315	322
6'0"	140	147	154	162	169	177	184	191	199	206	213	221	228	235	243	250	258	265	272	279	287	294	302	309	316	324	331
6'1"	144	151	159	166	174	182	189	197	204	212	219	227	235	242	250	257	263	272	280	288	295	302	310	318	325	333	340
6'2"	148	155	163	171	179	186	194	202	210	218	225	233	241	249	256	264	272	280	287	295	303	311	319	326	334	342	350
6'3"	152	160	168	176	184	192	200	208	216	224	232	240	248	256	264	272	279	287	295	303	311	319	327	335	343	351	359
6'4"	156	164	172	180	189	197	205	213	221	230	238	246	254	263	271	279	287	295	304	312	320	326	339	344	353	361	369

Instructions: Find your patient's height on the far left column, then move to the right to find the weight (lbs) in the corresponding row. Then ascend the column to determine the BMI. For instance, a woman who is 5'6" tall and weighs 229 lbs has a BMI of 37

> **Recommendations**
>
> All women with a BMI of > 30 should be counseled on the increased complications associated with pregnancy and delivery. Further, they should be encouraged to undergo dietary counseling and lose weight. Depending on the degree of the obesity, referral to a weight-loss specialist and screening for diabetes may be warranted. More aggressive management is needed for women with a BMI > 40 who should be strongly encouraged to lose weight prior to conceiving.

Caffeine intake

There have been several publications in the literature, which have demonstrated a dose-dependent relationship between caffeine intake and reduced fertility. Further, caffeine intake during pregnancy increases the chance of a spontaneous abortion and a low-birth-weight baby[27]. Therefore, it is reasonable to suggest to women who are attempting pregnancy to discontinue their caffeine intake, or at least, limit their intake to one caffeinated beverage a day. The quantity of caffeine in beverages is variable. The amount in a cup of coffee, tea and a can of soda is approximately 100, 50 and 50 mg, respectively. Men experience no fertility risk from caffeine intake. Interestingly, sperm exposed to caffeine-like drugs in the laboratory actually have enhanced motility.

Vitamin supplementation

Women who take folic acid prior to pregnancy have a reduced chance of having a baby with a neural tube defect. Neural tube defects are abnormal developments of the spine and skull. A common type of neural tube defect is spina bifida. In the United States, neural tube defects complicate 1 in 1000 deliveries. Previous studies have reported that women who supplemented their daily diet with 0.4 mg of folic acid experienced a 60–100% reduction in the frequency of neural tube defects[28-31]. After reviewing the available evidence, the US Public Health Service recommended the following:

> 'All women of child bearing age in the United States who are capable of becoming pregnant should consume 0.4 mg of folic acid per day for the purpose of reducing the risk of having a pregnancy affected with spina bifida or another neural tube defect.'

All women should be encouraged to follow these recommendations. This can be accomplished either through dietary supplementation or by taking an over-the-counter multivitamin preparation, which contains 0.4 mg of folic acid. Women who are overweight (BMI > 30) have an increased chance of having a baby with a neural tube defect[32]. In this population, it is prudent to prescribe a daily supplement of 1.0 mg of folic acid or a prenatal vitamin, which also contains 1.0 mg of folic acid. It is recommended that a woman who has had a previous pregnancy complicated by a neural tube defect or a family history of this defect should be treated with 4.0 mg of folic acid daily[33–35].

While vitamin supplementation is helpful, excessive vitamin intake can prove to be harmful to the developing fetus. Published data have confirmed that excessive intake of vitamin A increases the chance of congenital anomalies involving craniofacial, cardiac, thymus and central nervous system organ systems[36]. Isotretinoin (Accutane®), a derivative of vitamin A, is used to treat severe acne. In women who take this drug orally during pregnancy there is a 25% chance of congenital anomalies[37]. Prenatal vitamins and over-the-counter multivitamins contain 5000–8000 IU of vitamin A, which is a safe dose. However, daily intake of vitamin A should not exceed 10 000 IU. Excessive intake of animal liver, a food that is rich in vitamin A, should also be avoided. Supplementation with β-carotene, a precursor of vitamin A, is not associated with a toxic effect.

Recommendations for folic acid supplementation to prevent neural tube defects (NTD)*

- *Routine* – 0.4 mg daily (a multivitamin)

- *Obesity (BMI > 30)* – 1.0 mg daily (a prenatal vitamin or a 1.0 mg folic acid tablet)

- *Previous history or family history of NTD* – 4.0 mg folic acid daily[†]

*For adequate prevention of a NTD the folic acid supplement should be started 1 month before conception and continued during pregnancy.

[†]This level of intake can be achieved either by taking four 1.0 mg tablets of folic acid or three 1.0 mg folic acid tablets plus a prenatal vitamin. To achieve this level of supplementation more that one multivitamin (or prenatal vitamin) should ***not*** be taken on a daily basis. This will increase the intake of vitamin A over the safe level, which could increase the chances of birth defects.

Herbal remedies

Over the past several years, there has been increased use of alternative medical treatments including herbal remedies. Many of these herbal remedies are advertised as 'natural' and do not require a prescription. In a previous study, three commonly used herbs including St. John's Wort, *Echinacea purpura* and *Ginkgo biloba* were demonstrated to be detrimental to egg and sperm function[38]. Therefore, any woman who takes these medications should be encouraged to discontinue their use. Unfortunately, there are few published data on the hundreds of other herbal remedies. It is important to ask patients about the use of all medications, including herbal remedies. Many patients do not view herbal or over-the-counter medications as 'true' medications. Until published studies confirm the safety of herbal remedies, women should be encouraged to discontinue these agents before and after pregnancy is established.

ROUTINE GYNECOLOGICAL CARE

Every women should have a yearly blood pressure check, physical examination, pelvic examination and Pap smear. A baseline mammogram is recommended for every woman between the ages of 35 and 40 years. After the age of 40, a mammogram should be obtained every 1–2 years.

LABORATORY TESTING

Routine laboratory studies are an essential part of preconceptional care. Basically, the same tests that are routine for any pregnant woman should also be performed on the woman who is contemplating a pregnancy. The tests that we recommend are presented below. A complete blood count may identify a woman who has anemia or some other abnormality that needs attention. A blood type and screen may uncover the presence of an antibody that could increase the chance of isoimmunization. In addition, knowing the blood type is also advantageous when a patient is experiencing bleeding during the early part of pregnancy and the clinician needs to know whether anti-D immuno-globulin is indicated. Thyroid screening should be done with a serum TSH determination. Thyroid dysfunction is relatively common in the female population and can complicate a pregnancy. Since thyroid disorders can be genetic any woman who has a family history of thyroid dysfunction should be screened with antimicrosomal antibodies. Despite a normal TSH level, if a woman has positive antibodies she is at risk for thyroid problems in the future.

Certain infections during pregnancy can pose a health risk to the mother and/or fetus. During childhood it is public policy to administer immunizations that provide protection against many of these infections. Despite these efforts, a segment of the population remains at risk because of failure to receive the vaccine or failure to convert to immunity following a vaccination. Determining the immune status to certain infections including rubella, varicella and hepatitis should be considered a routine part of preconceptional care. Screening for other infectious diseases may be indicated depending on the clinical circumstances.

Preconceptional blood work

- TSH
- CBC
- Blood type & screen
- RPR
- Antibody screens for:
  – Rubella
  – Varicella
  – Hepatitis
  – HIV
- Genetic screening (if indicated)

Rubella (German measles)

Rubella is a self-limited viral infection that is associated with a characteristic rash. A maternal infection during the first trimester of pregnancy can result in fetal death or cause severe damage to cardiac, neurological, ophthamological and auditory organs. A major concern of a rubella infection is that almost one-third of infections are asymptomatic and, therefore, go undiagnosed. In the past, rubella was an endemic infection that affected our population. Since the introduction of the rubella vaccine in 1969, there has been a significant reduction in rubella infections and babies born with congenital rubella syndrome. However, despite these efforts, one in nine women are non-immune to rubella[39]. Screening for rubella immune status should be routinely performed on any woman who is contemplating pregnancy. Those women who are non-immune should be encouraged to receive the vaccine. The rubella vaccine is a live-attenuated virus and women should avoid pregnancy for 3 months after receiving the vaccine.

Varicella (chicken pox)

Varicella is a highly contagious viral infection that is caused by a herpes virus. Most individuals experience a memorable varicella infection during their childhood, which confers lifelong immunity. A non-immune individual can acquire the infection after exposure to an individual who has a primary varicella infection or herpes zoster (a latent form of varicella). Symptoms of an infection include malaise, fever and the development of characteristic vesicular lesions. Approximately 5% of individuals are non-immune to varicella[40]. There are concerns about a primary varicella infection that develops in an adult. Up to 20% of adults, who acquire a primary varicella infection will develop a concomitant pneumonia, which is fatal in 40% of cases[41]. If a pregnant woman develops the infection during the first trimester there is an increased incidence of congenital anomalies[40].

Immunity to varicella can be assessed by blood testing. A varicella vaccine is available and should be offered to non-immune individuals. The vaccine is administered in two doses 4–8 weeks apart. Because the varicella vaccine contains a live-attenuated virus, it is recommended that pregnancy be avoided during the vaccination and until 1 month after the last injection.

Hepatitis screening

There are six types of viral hepatitis (A, B, C, D, E and G). The severity and risk for vertical transmission varies depending on the type. Any woman who has been diagnosed with hepatitis in the past should receive counseling about the risks during pregnancy. Screening for hepatitis B is recommended for all pregnant women. Consideration should also be given to screening women as part of preconceptional care. While those with documented immunity to hepatitis pose no risk to the fetus, chronic carrier states do exist that can be associated with liver dysfunction and vertical transmission of the infection to the fetus. Women who have chronic active hepatitis B should be appropriately counseled and their infants at birth should receive HBIG to prevent an infection[42]. Individuals who work with blood products or who are at high risk for a hepatitis B infection should be offered immunization.

HIV testing

An HIV infection will lead to acquired immunodeficiency syndrome (AIDS). This viral infection targets and debilitates the immune system, which normally provides protection against infections. Many people who are infected with the virus continue to lead normal lives for some time, but eventually, (i.e. months to years after the initial infection) the immune system becomes more and more debilitated, serious symptoms develop and death results. Initially, the disease was found primarily in homosexual men, but the infection has been confirmed in the heterosexual population, as well. Many people who do not know that they are infected can infect others mainly through sexual contact. Of great concern, is that an asymptomatic woman who is infected with the virus can pass the infection to her unborn child. The course of the HIV infection in infants is the same as in adults. Because of the consequences of an HIV infection, it is strongly recommended that HIV testing be performed on all couples who are contemplating pregnancy.

MEDICAL HISTORY

An important aspect of preconceptional care is an in-depth medical history to identify medical problems that could complicate a pregnancy. A medical condition or the medications used to treat the condition can have an impact on the establishment and health of a pregnancy. Another concern is that the pregnancy can worsen the medical condition and impact on the health of the mother. In some cases, obtaining medical clearance may be indicated from the treating physician or a high-risk obstetrician before initiating treatment. Some of the more common medical problems that can be encountered are discussed below.

Diabetes mellitus

During pregnancy, diabetes mellitus is a commonly encountered medical problem. It has been estimated that approximately 6% of the general population and 3% of pregnant women are diabetic. Diabetes is associated with an increased incidence of congenital anomalies, which is directly related to the control of the diabetes prior to conception. A blood glucose level gives the clinician an idea of the glucose control at that point in time. The hemoglobin (Hgb) A1C level is a good indicator of how well the diabetes has been controlled over the previous 3–4 months. If the Hgb A1C is in the normal range then the incidence of congenital anomalies approaches the incidence in the general population. In addition to the increased risk of congenital anomalies, poorly controlled diabetes can be associated with increased fetal and maternal wastage. Therefore, the objective in the diabetic woman is to establish tight control of the glucose levels prior to conception. Vascular disease can complicate diabetes and warrants an assessment of renal function and an ophthalmological examination (to rule out a retinopathy) prior to pregnancy. There is also an increased incidence of pre-eclampsia in women with diabetes.

Screening for diabetes should be considered in a woman who is overweight (BMI > 27), has documented insulin resistance, a family history of diabetes, hypertension, chronic anovulation (PCO) or a previous pregnancy that was complicated by gestational diabetes or macrosomia. Screening for diabetes can be accomplished by a fasting plasma glucose test or the 75-g oral glucose tolerance test (which includes a fasting plasma glucose test and a 2-hour glucose determination). Fasting is defined as the intake of nothing more than water for a period of 8 hours. The American Diabetes Association interpretation of the glucose tolerance test is given in Table 2.1. Patients diagnosed with diabetes should be referred for further evaluation and treatment.

Hypertension

Chronic hypertension is a commonly encountered medical problem and, if left untreated, can cause irreparable damage to the kidneys and heart. Women with chronic hypertension should have baseline renal studies performed prior to conceiving. Hypertension places a woman at increased risk of superimposed pre-eclampsia during the pregnancy, even if it is well controlled. Presently, there are many types of medications that control hypertension. The adverse effects of any medication should be investigated to assess whether there are any adverse effects on a pregnancy.

Advanced maternal age

The current technology has increased the ability for women over the age of 40 years to achieve a pregnancy with egg donation. However, older women are at increased risk for complications during pregnancy as compared to their younger counterparts. With advancing age, every woman is at increased risk of developing diabetes mellitus, chronic hypertension and coronary artery disease,

Table 2.1 American Diabetes Association (ADA) threshold glucose values

Time	Normal	Borderline	Diabetes mellitus
Fasting	< 110 mg/dl	110–125 mg/dl	≥ 126 mg/dl
2 hours	< 140 mg/dl	140–199 mg/dl	≥ 200 mg/dl

For screening purposes it is recommended to do a fasting blood glucose initially. If the fasting blood glucose is abnormal then a 2-hour glucose tolerance test should be performed. For this test a fasting level is measured, the patient drinks 75 g of glucose and blood is drawn again 2 hours later for a glucose determination which can complicate a pregnancy. Therefore, it is prudent that every woman over the age of 42 undergoes a medical evaluation prior to undergoing treatment to assess her medical fitness for a pregnancy.

Medication use

All medications that a woman is taking should be investigated for potential detrimental effects on a pregnancy. The Food and Drug Administration (FDA) has placed medications into several categories based on animal and human studies that have investigated the harmful effects during pregnancy:

FDA drug categories for fetal toxicity

A   Adequate studies in pregnant women have failed to show a risk to the fetus in the first trimester of pregnancy and there is no evidence of risk in later trimesters.

B   Animal studies have not shown an adverse effect on the fetus, but there are no adequate clinical studies in pregnant women.

C   Animal studies have shown an adverse effect on the fetus, but there are no adequate studies in humans. The drug may be useful in pregnant women despite its potential risks.

D   There is evidence of risk to the human fetus, but the potential benefits of use in pregnant women may be acceptable despite potential risks.

X   Studies in animals or humans show fetal abnormalities, or adverse reaction reports indicate evidence of fetal risk. The risks involved clearly outweigh potential benefits.

It is clear that if a pregnant woman is taking a category X medication that it should be discontinued. However, if the medication falls into one of the other categories, continuation of the medication during pregnancy may be considered. Whether to continue the medication or not, is dependent on several factors. The first consideration is the nature and severity of the medical condition that is being treated. If the medical condition is not life-threatening or of significant importance, then serious consideration should be given to discontinuing the medication. In other situations, not treating the medical condition may put the mother or fetus at risk. In this situation, the clinician must try to select a medication that is effective in treating the condition and yet minimizes the risk to the fetus. For any medical therapy, if the benefits of treating the medical condition clearly outweigh the risks to the fetus then the medication should be continued. When making these decisions, it is important to have discussions with the patient and to obtain informed consent.

There are several resources to find information about the safety of any medication during pregnancy. The Physician's Desk Reference (PDR) is a good resource. Pharmacists have access to information that may be helpful. In addition, there are several internet resources which are presented below.

Internet resources for reproductive toxins

Pregnancy and Environmental Hotline
    http://www.thegenesisfund.org/hotline.htm
TOXLINE
    http://toxnet.nlm.nih.gov/cgi-bin/sis/htmlgen?TOXLINE
United States Food and Drug Administration
    http://www.fda.gov/cder/
Physicians Desk Reference
    www.pdr.net
Reprotox
    www.reprotox.org
TERIS & Shepard's Catalog of Teratogenic Agents
    http://depts.washington.edu/~terisweb/

REPRODUCTIVE HISTORY

A reproductive history is an important part of preconceptional care and the details of previous pregnancies should be obtained. If a woman has had a previous pregnancy with complications, she could be at increased risk for the recurrence of these complications with a future pregnancy. Therefore, any pregnancy with an abnormal outcome should be investigated before attempting pregnancy. The correction of an underlying problem may improve the outcome of a future pregnancy. Some of the more common issues concerning the reproductive history are discussed below.

Recurrent miscarriages

If a couple has experienced two or more miscarriages then an evaluation is indicated. A survey of lifestyle issues and environmental factors may give insight into the pregnancy losses. The work-up includes karyotypes on both the female and male partner to rule out chromosomal anomalies. A balanced translocation can be present in up to 6–8% of couples. A menstrual history is important to determine whether ovulatory dysfunction may be a contributing factor. The female partner should have an assessment of TSH level, glucose, lupus anticoagulant and anticardiolipin antibodies. An assessment of the uterine cavity should also be performed to rule out an anatomical reason for the pregnancy losses such as, uterine fibroids, Müllerian defects and DES changes. An examination of the uterine cavity can be accomplished by a hysterosalpingogram, sonohysterogram or a hysteroscopy.

Previous stillborn or infant born with congenital anomalies

In most cases, when a previous pregnancy has resulted in a stillbirth or a baby with birth defects, testing has been performed on the fetus and the couple has undergone counseling. However, if there is uncertainty about the depth or scope of the work-up then the couple should be referred to a high-risk obstetrician for a consultation to determine the risk with a future pregnancy.

History of premature labor

The causes of premature labor are varied and can be secondary to premature rupture of the membranes, an abnormal uterine cavity (secondary to uterine fibroids, a Müllerian defect and DES), chorioamnionitis or an incompetent cervix. A history of premature labor places a woman at increased risk of a similar occurrence with a future pregnancy. A pregnancy complicated with premature labor and a malpresentation increases the likelihood of a Müllerian anomaly, which has an incidence of 2–3% in the general population. A vaginal ultrasound and a hysterosalpingogram will help to determine whether there has been any abnormal development of the cavity. Painless dilatation prior to the delivery suggests the diagnosis of incompetent cervix. These women should be counseled on the benefits of a cervical cerclage with a future pregnancy. Finally, a multiple pregnancy should be avoided in women with a previous history of premature labor.

Gestational diabetes

If a woman has been diagnosed with gestational diabetes during a pregnancy she is at increased risk of the same occurrence during a future pregnancy. In addition, these women are at increased risk of developing adult onset diabetes during their lifetime (approximately 2–4% chance per year). For this reason, women with a history of gestational diabetes should be screened for glucose intolerance with a 2-hour glucose tolerance test. If diabetes is diagnosed then referral to a medical endocrinologist or a high-risk obstetrician would be in order prior to attempting pregnancy. Adequate control of diabetes before conception decreases the chance of congenital anomalies and complications during the pregnancy.

Severe pre-eclampsia

Pre-eclampsia complicates 6–8% of all pregnancies. In most cases, pre-eclampsia occurs during the first pregnancy and does not recur. However, severe pre-eclampsia that starts during the second trimester may recur in 10–15% of future pregnancies. It may be increased to a greater degree if there are any underlying risk factors including diabetes, renal dysfunction, chronic hypertension or a thrombophilia. Women with a history of severe pre-eclampsia may benefit from a referral to a high-risk obstetrician for counseling.

OCCUPATIONAL HISTORY

There is increased awareness about the impact of environmental toxic exposures on general and reproductive health. Toxic exposures at the work place can put some individuals at considerable risk. The Occupational Safety and Health Administration (OSHA), a federal agency of the Department of Labor, was established in 1970 and has monitored safety in the workplace. One of the three categories of hazardous substances monitored by the OSHA is reproductive toxins. Reproductive toxins are categorized as mutagens, teratogens, fertility toxins and toxins transferred at lactation. It has been estimated that 17% of working women are exposed to known teratogens in the workplace[43]. The following is a discussion of some occupational risks that may pose a risk to reproduction.

Exposure to anesthetic gases

It is well documented that women who are exposed to anesthetic gases (i.e. operating room personnel, dental hygentists) are at increased risk for infertility, spontaneous abortion and congenital anomalies[44–46]. Of interest is that paternal exposure may also be of consequence. Women who were impregnated by men who were exposed to anesthetic gases were found to be at greater risk of a having a pregnancy complicated by a spontaneous abortion and congenital anomalies[46].

Exposure to beauty salon chemicals

Beauty salon workers work in a complex environment and are exposed to many chemicals in hair dyes, permanent solutions and bleaches. Further, nail sculpturing also involves exposure to volatile chemicals that can be inhaled. A previous study concluded that beauty salon workers have an increased risk of miscarriage and infertility[47]. The risk was influenced by the number of hours worked per week, the use of formaldehyde disinfectants, the practice of using gloves during hair treatments and whether nail sculpturing was done in the salon.

Exposure to video display terminals

Many jobs require long hours in front of a video display terminal (VDT), or computer monitor. The theoretical concern over a VDT is that it creates an electromagnetic field. It is reassuring that studies have failed to associate VDT exposure with an increased risk of a spontaneous abortion and infertility[48,49].

Organic solvents

All women should be asked about exposure to organic solvents. Organic solvents include aliphatic and aromatic hydrocarbons, phenols, trichloroethylene, xylene, vinyl chloride and acetone. Women at greatest risk for exposure to these chemicals are those who work in the health-care profession, and the clothing and textile industries. However, women in other professions may be unknowingly exposed to these agents, as well. In a previous prospective study, women who were exposed to organic solvents during the first trimester were followed throughout the pregnancy[50]. When compared to a control group there was no statistical difference in the rate of a spontaneous abortion and minor malformations. However, the group exposed to organic solvents had a statistically higher incidence of major malformations when compared to controls (12% vs. 1%, $p < 0.001$).

Exposure to spermatotoxins

From a fertility standpoint, males are more susceptible to toxins since sperm production is an ongoing process. The first report of an occupationally related spermatotoxin appeared in the mid-1970s[51]. It showed that men who worked at factories which produced DBCP (a pesticide) had an increased incidence of infertility – the severity being dependent on the dose and length of exposure. Since this report was released, other spermatotoxins have been discovered including: kepone, ethylene glycol ethers, carbon disulfide, naphthyl methyl-carbamate, ethylene dibromide, organic solvents and lead.

Recommendation

As part of preconceptional care it is important to assess whether either the male or female partner are exposed to any toxin in the workplace that may prove detrimental. All employers must provide material safety data sheets (MSDS) of all chemicals that are present in the workplace. Any potential risk is dependent on the specific toxin, length of time of exposure and degree of exposure. If there is concern about an exposure, a consultation with a specialist in occupational medicine will help to clarify the risk.

GENETIC COUNSELING AND SCREENING

Advances in molecular biology and genetics have enhanced our understanding of the pathogenesis of disease. As our knowledge in the field of genetics expands an increasing responsibility will rest with those who counsel and prepare couples for pregnancy. A genetic history should be part of every evaluation of the infertile couple. There is no consensus as to the scope and breadth of the genetic history. Ideally, every couple contemplating a pregnancy would be evaluated by a geneticist or genetic counselor to determine their genetic risk. This obviously is not practical but some general assessment of genetic risk and counseling is indicated. A sample genetic screening is incorporated into our history forms (see Chapter 3).

It is important that any practitioner who is providing genetic counseling has an understanding of the disease process, its inheritance and the limitations of the screening tests that are currently available. In addition, it is of utmost importance that the clinician stays abreast of new clinical developments and screening tests that become available. If the practitioner is unable to adhere to this standard then referral to a genetic counselor would be appropriate. Recommendations for genetic counseling and position statements concerning testing have been published by the American College of Obstetrics and Gynecology (www.acog.com) and the American College of Medical Genetics (www.Faseb.org/genetics/acmg/acmgmenu.htm). An overview of some of the more common genetics issues follows.

Ancestral backgrounds

An important aspect of the genetic history is an exploration of the ancestral backgrounds of both partners. Historically, individuals of a specific ethnic population are more likely to reproduce with others from the same population. This gives an opportunity for the propagation and higher prevalence rate of certain genetic disorders within these populations. The diseases that are more prevalent in this inheritance pattern are autosomal recessive. In this inheritance pattern, carriers are asymptomatic of the disease and both partners must be carriers to be at risk (one in four chance) of having a child that could be affected by the disease.

Some of the commonly inherited conditions and indicated testing are discussed below. Many of these diseases can result in early death or significant morbidity. If an individual does not have an at-risk ancestral background but does have a family history of the disease, he/she should undergo screening (Table 2.2). It is also important that any individual who is identified to be a carrier of a genetic disease should be instructed to tell his/her siblings so that they too can undergo screening.

Table 2.2 Genetic testing based on ancestral backgrounds

Ancestral group	Disease	Screening test
Caucasian, Native American	cystic fibrosis*	DNA testing
French Canadian, Cajun	Tay-Sachs	assessment of hexosaminadase enzyme activity or DNA testing
Jewish	Canavan disease cystic fibrosis* Gaucher disease Tay-Sachs	DNA testing DNA testing DNA testing assessment of hexosaminadase enzyme activity or DNA testing
African, Asian, Cambodia, Caribbean, Central America, India, Indonesia, Laos, Malaysia, Mediterranean, Middle Eastern, Pakistan, Thailand, Turkey, Vietnam	hemoglobinopathies	CBC, Hgb electrophoresis

*It is impractical to screen for all cystic fibrosis mutations since over 900 mutations have been identified. Therefore, the clinician must realize the limitations of the screening and counsel couples accordingly. For instance, the detection rate of cystic fibrosis carriers in the Caucasian, Native American and Jewish populations is 90, 94 and 97%, respectively

Screening for chromosomal anomalies

In some situations, a chromosomal analysis may be indicated. The following are some indications in which a karyotype of the male and female partners may be indicated:

Recurrent miscarriages

Couples with two or more miscarriages have a 5–8% chance of having a balanced translocation. This chromosomal abnormality may explain the repeated miscarriages. While this chromosomal abnormality may put a couple at risk for a miscarriage, the majority of gametes that are produced in affected individuals are chromosomally normal. If a viable pregnancy is established when one of the partners has a balanced translocation there is concern that the fetus may have a chromosomal imbalance that would increase the risk of congenital anomalies. In these cases, the couple may consider genetic testing with chorionic villus sampling or a genetic amniocentesis.

History of Down's syndrome

If during the genetic history it is determined that a first-degree relative was diagnosed with Down's syndrome then it should be ascertained whether the affected individual underwent chromosomal testing. Approximately 90% of cases of Down's syndrome are trisomy 21 which is a sporadic event. The remaining 10% are the result of a translocation. Of these, half are inherited and the other half occur *de novo*. Therefore, if there is uncertainty about the etiology or the result of the chromosomal analysis of the affected individual with Down's syndrome then a karyotype should be offered.

History of a stillborn infant, congenital anomalies

In situations when a couple gives birth to a stillborn infant or an infant with a congenital anomaly, the chromosomal make-up of the fetus is usually tested. If this testing was not done or was inconclusive then chromosomal testing of the couple should be offered.

Severe male factor infertility

In males with severe oligospermia (< 5 million sperm/cc) there is a 6–8% chance of chromosomal anomalies and, therefore, these individuals should be offered chromosomal testing.

Fragile X screening

Mental retardation can be caused by many factors including environmental, social, genetic and unknown factors. The most commonly inherited type of mental retardation is Fragile X syndrome which affects 1 in 1200 males and 1 in 2500 females. Fragile X syndrome is the result of expansion of a repeat section on the long arm of the X chromosome. The degree of mental retardation can be borderline to severe and is associated with characteristic features including a long thin facies with prominent jaws, autistic features, and speech and language difficulties. Fragile X syndrome has an atypical inheritance. Some males who have the abnormal gene are unaffected while up to one-third of carrier females have associated mental retardation. For couples with a family history of unexplained mental retardation or autism, fragile X screening should be offered.

Maternal age counseling

Advanced maternal age is associated with an increased incidence of post-fertilization chromosomal abnormalities in the embryo. This explains why increased maternal age is associated with an increased incidence of infertility, pregnancy loss and an infant born with a chromosomal anomaly. While most pregnancies complicated by a chromosomal anomaly result in a miscarriage, others will progress to term resulting in a delivery. Therefore, advanced maternal age is a reason to offer a pregnant woman the option of prenatal genetic testing with a genetic amniocentesis or chorionic villus sampling. Following genetic testing, the most common chromosomal anomaly detected in the fetus is trisomy 21. However, there is also an increased incidence of trisomy 13 and trisomy 18 in addition to aneuploidy involving the sex chromosome including 47,XXY and 47,XXX. The incidence of fetal chromosomal anomalies according to maternal age is presented in Table 2.3.

Paternal age counseling

There is evidence that advanced paternal age can also pose a risk to the fetus, not on the basis of chromosomal abnormalities, but in the transmission of new genetic mutations. It is well established that older fathers are more likely to pass on new dominant inherited conditions to their children. In contrast to oogenesis, spermatogenesis is an ongoing process that continues throughout a man's life and it has been estimated that sperm stem cells divide 23 times each year. Assuming that this process is constant, by the time a man is 40 there will have been approximately 656 divisions (27 times the number of divisions that occur

Table 2.3 Chromosomal abnormalities in liveborn infants and maternal age*

Maternal age (years)	Risk for Down's syndrome	Total risk for chromosomal anomalies[†]
20	1/1667	1/526
21	1/1667	1/526
22	1/1429	1/500
23	1/1429	1/500
24	1/1250	1/476
25	1/1250	1/476
26	1/1176	1/476
27	1/1111	1/455
28	1/1053	1/435
29	1/1000	1/417
30	1/952	1/385
31	1/909	1/385
32	1/769	1/322
33	1/602	1/286
34	1/485	1/238
35	1/378	1/192
36	1/289	1/156
37	1/224	1/127
38	1/173	1/102
39	1/136	1/83
40	1/106	1/66
41	1/82	1/53
42	1/63	1/42
43	1/49	1/33
44	1/38	1/26
45	1/30	1/21
46	1/23	1/16
47	1/18	1/13
48	1/14	1/10
49	1/11	1/8

* The data presented above were modified from Hook DB, Cross PK, Schreinemachers DM. Chromosomal abnormality rates at amniocentesis and in live-born infants. *J Am Med Assoc* 1983; 249:2034–8, and Hook EB. Rates of chromosomal abnormalities at different maternal ages. *Obstet Gynecol* 1981;58:282–5

[†] The other chromosomal anomalies that are increased with maternal age in addition to 47,+21 (Down's syndrome) are 47,+18; and 47,+13; 47,XYY (Klinefelter's syndrome); 47,XYY and 47,XXX. The incidence of 47,XXX for women between the ages of 20 and 32 years is not available

in oocytes). The increased frequency of divisions increases the chance of errors that can result in a new mutation. This has been referred to as a 'copy error' which can result in the stem cells accumulating a mutation with each division. The incidence of the inheritance of an autosomal dominant condition is 1 in 5000–10 000 deliveries. While the paternal age effect on the occurrence of any specific autosomal dominant condition may be low, the combined effect on all autosomal dominant conditions can be significant. It has been estimated that a father at age 40 has at least a 0.3–0.5% chance of transmitting a dominant condition to the fetus. This is roughly the chance of a woman at age 35 of having a child with Down's syndrome.

While advanced paternal age increases the risk of these new mutations, testing for all of these dominantly inherited conditions is not possible. Further, there is no consensus as to the definition of advanced paternal age. It has been estimated that one-third of new autosomal dominant mutations are the result of advanced paternal age (> 40). It seems prudent to suggest that men complete their families by age 40. Even though there is no easy way to screen for all of these genetic conditions *in utero*, at the very least, couples should be made aware of the potential risk and given the opportunity to meet with a genetic counsellor.

CONCLUSION

Any couple who is interested in pregnancy should have a thorough evaluation to identify factors that may put the patient at risk for a complicated pregnancy. Depending on the situation, further work-up or counseling may be indicated before the couple attempts pregnancy.

3.
Accomplishing the work-up

The challenge for a clinician is how to accomplish the infertility evaluation in an organized and efficient manner. To this end, we have developed forms and narratives that help to achieve this goal. The documents included in this chapter of the handbook are for review and can be used in your clinical practice.

(1) **History forms**   The female and male history forms included are comprehensive and include an assessment of medical, social, environmental, genetic and occupational factors that are of importance. In addition, an extensive fertility history is also included in the history forms. These forms can be sent to the couple to be completed in advance of the consultation. The nurse/physician reviewing these forms can make additional notes in the comment section along the side of the forms. After the forms are filled out they can become part of the permanent medical record. These history forms were developed in part to support the documentation that is necessary for the CPT coding of consultation visits.

(2) **Preconceptional care narrative: things you must know before you get pregnant**   At the initial consultation, preconceptional issues should be discussed with the couple. As part of the process, the preconceptional narrative can be given to the couple for their review record.

(3) **Infertility evaluation narrative**   This form is given to the couple after the consultation. A notation or check mark can be made next to the tests that will be performed. Within the narrative there is a discussion of the rationale, performance and risks of the tests. Information is also provided for the patient regarding the scheduling of the tests. Consent forms for the infertility tests are also available in Chapter 10.

(4) **Infertility evaluation summary**   This sheet has a dual purpose. It can be used as an order form for the physician to check-off the tests that need to be done. In addition, the test results can be entered on this sheet which allows the physician to review all of the test results easily at the time of the follow-up consultation.

BOSTON IVF | FEMALE INTAKE FORM

TODAY'S DATE: ___/___/___
month day year

Patients – please complete all pages of this form.

NAME: _____ _____ AGE: _____ DOB:___/___/___
Last   First   month day year

OCCUPATION: _____

PARTNER'S NAME: _____ _____ AGE: _____ DOB:___/___/___
Last   First   month day year

REFERRING PHYSICIAN: _____ PRIMARY CARE PHYSICIAN: _____

ADDRESS _____ ADDRESS _____

PHONE NO.: _____ PHONE NO.: _____

MARITAL STATUS: ❒ Single   ❒ Separated   ❒ Divorced   ❒ Married _____ years

REASON FOR VISIT: _____

TRYING TO CONCEIVE?   ❒ No   ❒ Yes If so, how long without protection? _____ Years _____ months

Please answer the following questions. Do not write in shaded areas.

Menstrual History

Age you started to have periods	_____ yrs	
Are your periods regular?	❒ Yes ❒ No	
If cycles irregular, number cycles/year	_____ cycles	
On average, how many days between periods?	_____ days	
How long do your periods last?	_____ days	
Menstrual flow:	❒ Normal ❒ Light ❒ Heavy	
Pain with your periods?	❒ None ❒ Mild ❒ Mod ❒ Severe	
Pain not associated with your periods?	❒ Yes ❒ No	
Bleeding between periods?	❒ Yes ❒ No	
Date of last menstrual period	___/___/___	
Frequency of intercourse (per week)	_____	

Comments:

Gynecological History

Gonorrhea	❒ Yes ❒ No	Chlamydia	❒ Yes ❒ No
Pelvic infection	❒ Yes ❒ No	Herpes	❒ Yes ❒ No
Painful sex	❒ Yes ❒ No	Excessive hair	❒ Yes ❒ No
Breast discharge	❒ Yes ❒ No	Prior IUD use	❒ Yes ❒ No
Birth control pill	❒ Yes ❒ No	Mom took DES	❒ Yes ❒ No
Vaginal lubricants	❒ Yes ❒ No	Douche	❒ Yes ❒ No
Sexual abuse	❒ Yes ❒ No	Physical abuse	❒ Yes ❒ No
Abnormal Pap	❒ Yes ❒ No	Mammogram	❒ Yes ❒ No
Date last Pap: ___/___/___		Acne	❒ Yes ❒ No

Obstetric History

Date *(mo/yr)* Outcome *(circle one)*   *Comments/Complications?*

___/___ Miscar/Nml deliv/Cesar/Tubal/Abortion _____

___/___ Miscar/Nml deliv/Cesar/Tubal/Abortion _____

___/___ Miscar/Nml deliv/Cesar/Tubal/Abortion _____

___/___ Miscar/Nml deliv/Cesar/Tubal/Abortion _____

Prior Infertility Evaluation (if applicable)

		Year	Result	
Basal temp records	❏ No	____	❏ Normal	❏ Abnormal
Urine ovulation kits	❏ No	____	❏ Normal	❏ Abnormal
Endometrial biopsy	❏ No	____	❏ Normal	❏ Abnormal
Semen analysis	❏ No	____	❏ Normal	❏ Abnormal
Hysterosalpingogram	❏ No	____	❏ Normal	❏ Abnormal
Postcoital test	❏ No	____	❏ Normal	❏ Abnormal
Laparoscopy	❏ No	____	❏ Normal	❏ Abnormal
Hysteroscopy	❏ No	____	❏ Normal	❏ Abnormal
FSH blood test	❏ No	____	❏ Normal	❏ Abnormal

Prior Infertility Treatments (if applicable)

			Year	
Clomid or Serophene	❏ No	❏ Yes:	____	# cycles _____
FSH injectable meds.	❏ No	❏ Yes:	____	# cycles _____
hCG injectable med.	❏ No	❏ Yes:	____	# cycles _____
Intrauterine insemin.	❏ No	❏ Yes:	____	# cycles _____
IVF or GIFT	❏ No	❏ Yes:	____	# cycles _____

Take Medications   ❏ Yes   ❏ No

If yes, which ones: _____

_____

Do you take folic acid or vitamins?   ❏ Yes   ❏ No

Do you take herbal remedies?   ❏ Yes   ❏ No

Allergies   ❏ Yes   ❏ No

If yes, describe: _____

_____

What is your blood type?   ❏ Unknown   ❏ Blood type _____

Past Surgeries   ❏ Yes   ❏ Yes

If yes, state type, date, hospital:

_____

_____

_____

_____

Social

Smoke	❏ Yes ❏ No	Alcohol weekly	❏ Yes ❏ No
Cocaine	❏ Yes ❏ No	Marijuana	❏ Yes ❏ No
IV drugs	❏ Yes ❏ No	Weight change	❏ Yes ❏ No
Regular exercise	❏ Yes ❏ No	Caffeine	❏ Yes ❏ No

Comments:

Family History

Has anybody in your family had any of the following?

Early menopause	❏ Yes ❏ No	Breast cancer	❏ Yes ❏ No
Ovarian cancer	❏ Yes ❏ No	Muscular dystrophy	❏ Yes ❏ No
Stillbirth	❏ Yes ❏ No	Sickle-cell anemia	❏ Yes ❏ No
Cystic fibrosis	❏ Yes ❏ No	Mental retardation	❏ Yes ❏ No
Tay-Sachs	❏ Yes ❏ No	Spina bifida	❏ Yes ❏ No
Down's syndrome	❏ Yes ❏ No	Tuberous sclerosis	❏ Yes ❏ No
Birth defects	❏ Yes ❏ No	Heart attack (< 50 yrs)	❏ Yes ❏ No
Thyroid disease	❏ Yes ❏ No	Psychiatric disease	❏ Yes ❏ No
Diabetes	❏ Yes ❏ No	Blindness	❏ Yes ❏ No
High blood press.	❏ Yes ❏ No	Chromosome problem	❏ Yes ❏ No
Hemophilia	❏ Yes ❏ No	Recurrent miscarriage	❏ Yes ❏ No
Deafness	❏ Yes ❏ No	Other genetic disorders:	❏ Yes ❏ No
Polycystic kidneys	❏ Yes ❏ No	_____	
Bleeding disorders	❏ Yes ❏ No	_____	

Ancestral Background

There are certain ancestral backgrounds that have an increased frequency of some genetic diseases. Please indicate if either your mother or father are of any of the following backgrounds:

❏ African ❏ Caribbean ❏ Jewish ❏ Indian ❏ Native American
❏ French-Canadian ❏ Latin-American ❏ Mediterranean ❏ Asian

Medical History (Review of Systems)

Have you ever had any of the following?

Abdominal pains	❏ Yes ❏ No	Epilepsy	❏ Yes ❏ No
Anemia	❏ Yes ❏ No	Excessive thirst	❏ Yes ❏ No
Antibiotics	❏ Yes ❏ No	Fainting	❏ Yes ❏ No
Appendicitis	❏ Yes ❏ No	Fibroids	❏ Yes ❏ No
Arthritis	❏ Yes ❏ No	Exces. Constipation	❏ Yes ❏ No
Asthma	❏ Yes ❏ No	Severe headaches	❏ Yes ❏ No
Blood clots	❏ Yes ❏ No	Urinary infections	❏ Yes ❏ No
Blood in stool	❏ Yes ❏ No	Heart disease	❏ Yes ❏ No
Blood transfusion	❏ Yes ❏ No	Heat/cold intolerance	❏ Yes ❏ No
Problem with vision	❏ Yes ❏ No	Hepatitis, liver prob.	❏ Yes ❏ No
Breast discharge	❏ Yes ❏ No	High blood pressure	❏ Yes ❏ No
Cancer	❏ Yes ❏ No	Hot flashes, sweats	❏ Yes ❏ No
Diabetes	❏ Yes ❏ No	Lack bladder control	❏ Yes ❏ No
Dizziness	❏ Yes ❏ No	Anxiety	❏ Yes ❏ No
Easy bruising	❏ Yes ❏ No	Kidney problems	❏ Yes ❏ No
Endometriosis	❏ Yes ❏ No	Mitral valve prolapse	❏ Yes ❏ No
Neck/back pain	❏ Yes ❏ No	Thrombophlebitis	❏ Yes ❏ No
Neurological prob.	❏ Yes ❏ No	Thyroid problem	❏ Yes ❏ No
Nose/gum bleeds	❏ Yes ❏ No	Tuberculosis	❏ Yes ❏ No
Palpitations	❏ Yes ❏ No	Shortness of breath	❏ Yes ❏ No
Stomach problems	❏ Yes ❏ No	Swollen joints	❏ Yes ❏ No
German measles	❏ Yes ❏ No	Chicken pox	❏ Yes ❏ No

Comments:

BOSTON IVF **FEMALE INTAKE CLINICIAN'S ASSESSMENT**

TODAY'S DATE: ___/___/___
month day year

NAME: _____ _____ AGE: _____ DOB:___/___/___
Last   First   month day year

PHYSICIAN: _____

NURSE'S COMMENTS: _____

_____

_____

_____

_____

NURSE'S SIGNATURE: _____

Physical Exam

BP: ___/___   Pulse: _____   Height: _____ inches   Weight: _____ lbs   BMI: _____

HEENT	❐ Normal	❐ Abnormal: _____
LUNGS	❐ Clear	❐ Abnormal: _____
THYROID	❐ Normal	❐ Abnormal: _____
HEART	❐ Normal	❐ Abnormal: _____
BREASTS	❐ Normal	❐ Abnormal: _____
ABDOMEN	❐ Normal	❐ Abnormal: _____
EXTREM	❐ Normal	❐ Abnormal: _____

Pelvic

Vulva	❐ Normal	❐ Abnormal: _____
Cervix	❐ Normal	❐ Abnormal: _____
Uterus position	❐ AV ❐ RV	❐ AX
Uterus size	❐ Normal	❐ Abnormal: _____
Left adnexa	❐ Normal	❐ Abnormal: _____
Right adnexa	❐ Normal	❐ Abnormal: _____
Rectal	❐ Normal	❐ Abnormal: _____

Other Comments on Physical Exam

_____

_____

_____

_____

_____

_____

_____

Assessment/Plan

_____
_____
_____
_____
_____
_____
_____
_____
_____
_____
_____
_____
_____
_____
_____
_____
_____
_____
_____
_____
_____
_____
_____
_____
_____
_____
_____
_____
_____
_____
_____
_____
_____

Diagnosis

❒ Infertility – being evaluated	❒ Abortion – spontaneous	❒ Endometriosis	❒ PCO/Anov (no infertility)
❒ Infertility – male	❒ Adhesions	❒ Fibroid uterus	❒ Pelvic inflammatory disease
❒ Infertility – tubal factor	❒ Adnexal mass	❒ Hirsutism/hyperandrogen	❒ Postmenopausal bleeding
❒ Infertility – tubal occlusion	❒ Asherman's syndrome	❒ Hyperprolactonemia	❒ Pregnancy
❒ Infertility – unexplained	❒ Breast mass	❒ Menopausal	❒ Premature ovarian failure
❒ Infertility – immunological	❒ Cervical dysplasia	❒ Menopause – premature	❒ Premenstrual symptoms
❒ Infertility – anovulation	❒ DES in utero exposure	❒ Menstrual irregularity	❒ Urinary tract infection
❒ Infertility – cervical factor	❒ Dysfunctional bleeding	❒ Mullerian abnormality	❒ Vaginitis
❒ Abdominal/pelvic pain	❒ Dysmenorrhea	❒ Normal GYN	❒ Other: _____
❒ Abortion – recurrent	❒ Ectopic pregnancy	❒ Ovarian cyst	_____

BOSTON IVF | **MALE INTAKE FORM**

TODAY'S DATE: ____/____/____
month day year

NAME: _____ _____ AGE: _____ DOB: ____/____/____
    Last   First   month day year

PARTNER'S NAME: _____ _____ AGE: _____ DOB: ____/____/____
                 Last   First   month day year

REFERRING PHYSICIAN: _____ PRIMARY CARE PHYSICIAN: _____

REASON FOR VISIT: ❒ Infertility ❒ Other _____

IF TRYING TO CONCEIVE, HOW LONG? ❒ Yes _____ years   OCCUPATION _____

Please answer the following questions on the front and back of this page. Make any comments in the comments section at the bottom of this page.

Number of pregnancies with current partner: _____

Number of years married: _____ years

Number of prior marriages: Husband: ____ Wife: ____

Number of pregnancies with previous partner(s): ____

Age(s) of children, if any: _____

Past Medical History

Do you have any heart problems?   ❒ Yes ❒ No

Do you have any lung problems
  (asthma, etc.)?   ❒ Yes ❒ No

Do you have bowel or stomach
  problems?   ❒ Yes ❒ No

Problems with muscles or joints?   ❒ Yes ❒ No

Ever had mumps?   ❒ Yes ❒ No

Do you have any neurological problems? ❒ Yes ❒ No

Any hormonal problems
  (thyroid, diabetes, etc.)?   ❒ Yes ❒ No

Do you have any other medical problems?

_____

_____

_____

Have you had any other surgery?

_____

_____

List medications you are now taking:

_____

_____

ALLERGY to medications: ❒ Yes   ❒ No _____

Urological History

Have you ever had undescended testicles? ❒ Yes ❒ No

Have you ever suffered an injury to the testicles? ❒ Yes ❒ No

Have you ever had a hernia repair? ❒ Yes ❒ No

Have you been diagnosed with a varicocele? ❒ Yes ❒ No

Have you had a vasectomy? ❒ Yes ❒ No

Have you had bladder or prostate surgery? ❒ Yes ❒ No

Do you have a problem with achieving erections? ❒ Yes ❒ No

Have you had epididymitis? ❒ Yes ❒ No

Ever had a urinary tract infection? ❒ Yes ❒ No

Ever had a sexually transmitted disease? ❒ Yes ❒ No

Any problems with ejaculation? ❒ Yes ❒ No

Any problems with sex drive? ❒ Yes ❒ No

Did you have early puberty (before 12 yrs)? ❒ Yes ❒ No

Did you have late puberty? ❒ Yes ❒ No

Have you had abnormal sexual development? ❒ Yes ❒ No

Have you had a fever within the last 3 months? ❒ Yes ❒ No

Other family member have a fertility problem? ❒ Yes ❒ No

Social

Any special exposure to heat on a regular
  basis (sauna, baths, Jacuzzi)? ❒ Yes ❒ No

Do you use recreational drugs? ❒ Yes ❒ No

Do you smoke? ❒ Yes ❒ No

Have you been exposed to any chemicals? ❒ Yes ❒ No

Have you been exposed to radiation
  (not routine x-rays)? ❒ Yes ❒ No

How many drinks of alcohol per week? _____

_____

Comments on any of the above:

_____

_____

_____

Family History
Has anybody in your family had any of the following?

Breast cancer	❐ Yes	❐ No	Stillbirth	❐ Yes	❐ No	Tuberous sclerosis	❐ Yes	❐ No
Cystic fibrosis	❐ Yes	❐ No	Muscular dystrophy	❐ Yes	❐ No	Tay-Sachs	❐ Yes	❐ No
Sickle-cell anemia	❐ Yes	❐ No	Down's syndrome	❐ Yes	❐ No	Mental retardation	❐ Yes	❐ No
Birth defects	❐ Yes	❐ No	Spina bifida	❐ Yes	❐ No	Thyroid disease	❐ Yes	❐ No
High blood press.	❐ Yes	❐ No	Diabetes	❐ Yes	❐ No	Heart attack (< 50 yrs)	❐ Yes	❐ No
Blindness	❐ Yes	❐ No	Psychiatric disease	❐ Yes	❐ No	Hemophilia	❐ Yes	❐ No
Polycystic kidneys	❐ Yes	❐ No	Deafness	❐ Yes	❐ No	Chromosome problem	❐ Yes	❐ No
Ovarian cancer	❐ Yes	❐ No	Bleeding disorders	❐ Yes	❐ No	Other genetic disorders	❐ Yes	❐ No

Ancestral Background
There are certain ancestral backgrounds that have an increased frequency of some genetic diseases. Please indicate if either your mother or father are of any of the following backgrounds:

❐ African ❐ Caribbean ❐ Jewish ❐ Indian ❐ Native American ❐ French-Canadian ❐ Latin-American ❐ Mediterranean ❐ Asian

This section to be completed by your Physician

Laboratory Results

Semen Analysis	*Date*	*Date*	*Date*	*Other test results*
COUNT	_____	_____	_____	FSH _____
MOTILITY	_____	_____	_____	LH _____
MORPHOLOGY	_____	_____	_____	PRL _____
VOLUME	_____	_____	_____	TESTO/FT _____
Other Comments	_____	_____	_____	TSH _____

Physical Examination

GENERAL		❐ Normal	❐ Abnl:	_____
ABDOMEN		❐ Normal	❐ Abnl:	_____
PENIS		❐ Normal	❐ Abnl:	_____
Meatus		❐ Normal	❐ Abnl:	_____
TESTES	Left	❐ Normal	❐ Abnl:	_____
	Right	❐ Normal	❐ Abnl:	_____
VASA	Left	❐ Normal	❐ Abnl:	_____
	Right	❐ Normal	❐ Abnl:	_____
EPID	Left	❐ Normal	❐ Abnl:	_____
	Right	❐ Normal	❐ Abnl:	_____
PROSTATE		❐ Normal	❐ Abnl:	_____
VARICO	Left	❐ No	❐ Mild	❐ Mod ❐ Large
	Right	❐ No	❐ Mild	❐ Mod ❐ Large
Other Findings:		_____		
U/A:	Dip	❐ Normal	❐ Abnl:	_____
	PH:	_____		

Impression and Plan

_____

_____

_____

_____

_____

PRECONCEPTIONAL CARE: THINGS YOU MUST KNOW BEFORE YOU GET PREGNANT

We have two goals for your treatment. The first goal is to help you achieve a pregnancy. The second goal is that the pregnancy is uncomplicated and results in the delivery of a healthy baby. To this end, there are certain things that *you* can do to help achieve this goal, which are discussed below.

Smoking

The detrimental effects of smoking on general health are well established (e.g. heart disease, cancer and chronic lung disease). Smoking also impacts on reproductive health. Women who smoke during pregnancy are at increased risk for premature labor, decreased fetal growth and other complications. In addition, studies have demonstrated that men and women who smoke have a decreased chance of achieving a pregnancy either naturally or following infertility treatment. Therefore, if you smoke, we feel strongly that for general and reproductive health concerns, you must stop. If you are unable to stop on your own then you should contact your primary-care physician to get enrolled in a smoking cessation program.

Alcohol

Alcohol should be completely avoided during pregnancy because it increases the chance of the birth defects. In addition, alcohol can interfere with the establishment of pregnancy. A recent study concluded that any amount of alcohol ingested by the woman decreased the chance of pregnancy and increased the chance of a miscarriage. Therefore, we recommend that if a woman is attempting pregnancy she should completely avoid alcohol or limit intake to the first week of the menstrual cycle. There is no detriment of mild-to-moderate alcohol intake on male fertility.

Caffeine intake

Several studies have concluded that caffeine intake by the woman decreases the chance of establishing a pregnancy and increases the chance of a miscarriage. Caffeine is present in coffee, tea, soft drinks and chocolate. It is our recommendation that the woman should avoid caffeine altogether or limit intake to one caffeinated beverage per day. Decaffeinated beverages are safe. There is no detrimental effect of caffeine on male fertility.

Recreational drug use

The use of recreational drugs is absolutely contraindicated while attempting to conceive and during pregnancy. Some drugs, such as marijuana, may decrease sperm production. Drug use by the woman during pregnancy, such as cocaine and heroine, may lead to severe withdrawal reactions in the baby following birth. Further, the use of intravenous drugs increases the risk of acquiring an HIV and hepatitis infection.

Medication use

All non-fertility medications that have been prescribed should be discussed with your physician. It is also important that you contact the physician who originally prescribed these medications to make sure that he/she is aware that you are attempting pregnancy. You should avoid taking aspirin and aspirin-like compounds (e.g. Advil®, Aleve®, Ibuprofen® and Motrin®) around the time of ovulation, since these medications can interfere with ovulation. Tylenol® is a suitable alternative. Herbal remedies should be completely avoided since their effect on fertility and pregnancy are unknown.

Vitamin supplementation

Neural tube defects are birth defects that result in abnormal development of the spine and skull. One type of neural tube defect is spina bifida. Several studies have confirmed that folic acid supplementation started before conception will reduce the occurrence of neural tube defects in infants. It is now recommended that all women who are attempting pregnancy ingest at least 0.4 mg of folic acid per day for this protection. Folic acid supplementation can be achieved by taking an over-the-counter multivitamin or a prenatal vitamin on a daily basis.

There are published data that have confirmed that excessive intake of vitamin A increases the chance of congenital anomalies. Prenatal vitamins and over-the-counter multivitamins contain 5000 IU of vitamin A, which is a safe dose. However, daily intake should *not* exceed 10 000 IU.

HIV testing

An HIV infection can lead to the development of acquired immunodeficiency syndrome (AIDS). This viral infection targets and debilitates the immune system, which provides us protection against infection. Many people who are infected with the virus continue to lead normal lives for some time before developing symptoms. Of great concern is that many people who do not know that they are infected can infect others through sexual contact. A woman who is infected with the virus can pass the infection to her unborn child. The course of the HIV infection in infants is the same as in adults. Because of the consequences of an HIV infection, we recommend HIV testing for all couples contemplating pregnancy.

Exercise

The benefits of exercise on general health and mental well-being are established. Further, exercise during pregnancy has also been shown to be beneficial. If you are already in an exercise program, we would encourage you to continue. However, the medications used to stimulate the ovaries as part of your treatment can cause temporary ovarian cysts to form. Therefore, we would advise yo u to avoid exercise activities that result in a lot of vertical movement (i.e. running, step aerobics, etc.). Exercise activities such as swimming, bicycle riding, walking and using the treadmill or step exercise are acceptable.

Nutrition

Our general health is influenced by what we eat, how much we eat and how much energy we expend with activity and exercise. In addition, our nutritional state can impact on reproductive health, as well, and can influence the establishment and maintenance of a pregnancy. Extremes of body weight can be associated with altered ovarian function. As a general recommendation, women should be encouraged to maintain a balanced diet of fruits, vegetables, breads, meats and dairy products. Foods with a high content of fats and oils should be used at a minimum. In addition to a balanced diet, caloric intake should be limited to maintain a normal body weight.

Body weight

A major concern about increased weight is the higher chance of complications during pregnancy including diabetes, high blood pressure and clot formation. Women who are overweight tend to have larger babies, more difficult deliveries and a higher chance of requiring a Cesarean section. Furthermore, a Cesarean section that is performed on a woman who is overweight is associated with a higher incidence of anesthetic and surgical complications that could jeopardize the health of the mother and baby.

The body mass index (BMI) is a standard to determine whether a person's weight is appropriate for their height. It is a calculation that takes into account the weight and height [BMI = weight (kg)/height (m^2)]. An easy way to calculate the BMI is as follows: multiply the weight in pounds by 704 then divide by height (in inches) squared.

Example For a woman 5′ (60″) tall and weighing 207 lbs, her BMI would be calculated as follows:

$$207 \times 704/60^2 = 40.5$$

A woman is considered *normal* if the BMI is 20–24; *overweight* if the BMI is 25–29, *significantly overweight* if the BMI is 30–39, and *extremely overweight* if the BMI is 40 or higher.

Recommendations

All women with a BMI of > 30 should be encouraged to lose weight and a referral to a nutritionist, weight-loss specialist and/or a high-risk obstetrician may be recommended. Because of the associated risks, infertility treatment may be unsafe and contraindicated in women with a BMI > 40.

Routine gynecological care

During your infertility treatment, it is important for you to continue your routine follow-up with your gynecologist or primary-care physician. This should include a yearly blood pressure check, physical examination, pelvic examination and Pap smear. A baseline mammogram is recommended for every woman aged 35–40. After the age of 40, every woman should have a mammogram every 1–2 years.

THE INFERTILITY EVALUATION

The infertility evaluation consists of a series of tests that evaluates male and female reproductive function. The objective of the evaluation is to identify potential causes of infertility. Accordingly, your doctor may order any or all of the following tests, as it is important that a complete evaluation be performed. To help familiarize you with these tests and what can be learned from them, a description of each appears below.

☐ **Semen analysis**

The semen analysis is the standard test for the evaluation of the male partner. The semen analysis includes an assessment of the sperm concentration, motility (or activity of sperm) and a determination of the percentage of normally shaped sperm. If the initial semen analysis is found to be abnormal, then a repeat analysis may be requested.

Scheduling

We will instruct you on how to set up an appointment for the test.
Please read carefully and follow these instructions. If you have any questions, feel free to discuss them with us.

(1) The physician should be informed of all medications that you are taking.

(2) Exposure of the testes to high temperatures (saunas, hot baths) should be avoided since this will decrease the sperm count.

(3) You should abstain from ejaculation for 24 hours before the test. Decreasing the frequency of ejaculation '*to save sperm*' does not improve the results of the semen analysis.

(4) The specimen is produced by masturbation into a sterile container that will be provided. The sample can be produced at the laboratory or at home then brought in immediately. For the latter, the specimen should arrive at the laboratory no later than 30 minutes after it is produced. During transport, the specimen should be kept at body temperature and not exposed to extreme heat or cold. If the sample is to be produced at home, a container to collect the sample will be provided.

The results of the analysis will be discussed with you at the follow-up consultation or you will receive a letter from your physician. If for any reason the test must be repeated, you will be contacted.

☐ **Hormone testing of ovarian function**

An important factor that influences a woman's fertility is the number and quality of eggs, which can be assessed by hormone testing. Between days 2 and 4 of the menstrual cycle, a blood sample can be obtained for the measurement of follicle stimulating hormone (FSH) and estradiol hormones. FSH is made by the pituitary gland (located at the base of the brain). FSH stimulates the development of ovarian follicles, which are the fluid-filled cysts that contain the eggs. Estradiol is an estrogen hormone, which is produced by the developing follicle. An elevation in the FSH and/or estradiol levels suggests a reduction in the supply of eggs within the ovaries. In this circumstance, there may be a reduced chance of achieving pregnancy and an increased chance of a miscarriage if pregnancy is established.

Scheduling

On the first day of your menstrual period (cycle day 1) contact your physician's office and arrange for the blood test, which can be performed between cycle days 2 and 4. If your period occurs on the weekend, please call first thing Monday morning to schedule the test.

☐ Hysterosalpingogram (HSG)

A hysterosalpingogram (also called tubogram or hysterogram) is an X-ray that is performed to examine the uterine cavity and determine whether the Fallopian tubes are open.

Scheduling

On the first day of your menstrual period (cycle day 1) contact your physician's office to schedule the test. If your period occurs on the weekend, please call Monday morning to schedule the test. The test is performed in a radiologist's office and usually done between cycle days 5 and 12.

Performance of the test

First, a speculum is placed in the vagina to visualize the cervix. A small tube is then placed into the cervical canal. An iodine-containing fluid is injected gently through this tube into the uterine cavity. The progress of the dye is followed by viewing a television monitor. Generally, the test is completed within 4–5 minutes and is sometimes associated with temporary lower abdominal cramping which resolves after completion of the test. *You may benefit from taking two to three 200-mg tablets of ibuprofen (Advil®, Motrin®) 1 hour before your test.*

The complication rate from this procedure is less than 2%. Some of the risks include the following:

Pelvic infection The performance of this test can result in an infection that could produce lower abdominal pain and fever. A consequence of this infection may be scarred Fallopian tubes and infertility. An infection is more likely to occur in women who already have damaged Fallopian tubes.

Allergic reaction The contrast medium used contains iodine. *If you have had any allergic reaction to iodine, a reaction following another radiological procedure (e.g. CT scans, IVP) or if you have had a reaction to fish or shellfish, please notify your physician.* This could be suggestive of an iodine allergy.

Exposure to potential pregnancy Please notify your physician if you feel that your previous menstrual period was not normal. In this circumstance a pregnancy test can be done before the procedure.

Upon completion of the test the results will be discussed with you. Following the X-ray you are ready to resume your normal activities and can return to work. A discharge of clear fluid and vaginal spotting may be noted for the next day. You should refrain from intercourse for 2 days.

☐ Sonohysterogram

The sonohysterogram is a test that examines the uterine cavity and is sometimes done in lieu of or in conjunction with the hysterosalpingogram.

Scheduling

On the first day of your menstrual period (cycle day 1) contact your physician's office to schedule the test. If your period occurs on the weekend, please call Monday morning to schedule the test. The test is usually done between cycle days 5 and 12.

Performance of the test

First, a speculum is placed in the vagina to visualize the cervix. A small catheter is then placed through the cervical canal into the uterine cavity. The vaginal ultrasound probe is inserted into the vagina. Once the uterus is brought into view, a saline solution is injected into the cavity through the catheter. Generally, the test is completed within 4–5 minutes. The test is

sometimes associated with lower abdominal cramping. *You may benefit from taking two to three 200-mg tablets of ibuprofen (Advil, Motrin) 1 hour before your test.*

The complication rate from this procedure is less that 2%. Some of the risks include the following:

Pelvic infection The performance of this test can result in an infection that could produce lower abdominal pain and fever. A consequence of this infection may be scarred Fallopian tubes and infertility. An infection is more likely to occur in women who already have damaged Fallopian tubes.

Exposure to potential pregnancy Please notify your physician if you feel that your previous menstrual period was not normal. In this circumstance, a pregnancy test can be done before the procedure.

Upon completion of the test the results will be discussed with you. Following the test you are ready to resume your normal activities and can return to work. A discharge of clear fluid and vaginal spotting may be noted for the next day. You should refrain from intercourse for 2 days.

☐ Endometrial biopsy

An endometrial biopsy is an office procedure that involves the removal of a small amount of tissue from the uterine cavity. A pathologist will then examine the biopsy. Any woman who has a history of abnormal bleeding, irregular or absence of menstrual periods or a history of a biopsy confirming an infection may benefit from the performance of an endometrial biopsy. The endometrial biopsy *is not a routine test* and is done in selected cases.

Scheduling

Your physician will discuss with you the appropriate timing of the biopsy.

Performance of the test

First, a speculum is placed in the vagina to visualize the cervix. A small plastic catheter is placed into the cervical canal into the uterine cavity. The biopsy is obtained with this catheter. Generally, the biopsy is completed within a few minutes. The test is associated with some lower cramping. *You may benefit from taking two to three 200-mg tablets of ibuprofen (Advil, Motrin) 1 hour before your test.*

The complication rate from this procedure is less that 2%. Some of the risks include the following:

Pelvic infection The performance of this test can result in an infection that could produce lower abdominal pain and fever. A consequence of this infection may be scarred Fallopian tubes and infertility. An infection is more likely to occur in women who already have damaged Fallopian tubes.

Exposure to potential pregnancy P l e a s e notify your physician if you feel that your previous menstrual period was not normal. In this circumstance a pregnancy test can be done before the procedure.

You are ready to resume your normal activities and may return to work 1 hour after the endometrial biopsy is performed. Results should be available 1 week after the performance of the biopsy.

☐ **Surgery**

Laparoscopy

This is an outpatient surgical procedure that is performed under general anesthesia. This procedure involves the placement of a telescopic instrument through a small incision and into the abdominal cavity, which allows the visualization of the pelvic organs. The objective of the laparoscopy is to identify and treat any conditions involving pelvic organs (i.e. endometriosis, adhesions) that might be playing a role in your infertility. Following the surgery, you will need to be transported home. Usually, you are ready to return to normal activities approximately 2–3 days after the surgery.

Hysteroscopy

This is an outpatient surgical procedure. It can be performed by itself but many times is done in conjunction with a laparoscopy. The procedure involves the placement of a telescope through the cervical canal and into the uterine cavity. The cavity is distended with saline and then examined. The objective of this procedure is to identify and treat conditions in the uterine cavity (i.e. endometrial polyps and fibroids) that might be contributing to your infertility. Following the surgery, you will need to be transported home. Usually, you are ready to return to normal activities the day after your surgery.

□ **Counseling**

Dealing with infertility can be stressful. To help you deal with the stress, we can refer you to a social worker who has experience with infertile couples. Most psychological services are covered under the mental health benefit section of insurance plans. Please check with your insurance company regarding your benefits.

□ **Medical records**

Review of medical records from previous testing and treatment will help in the development of a treatment plan. Please obtain the following records:

□ *Hysterosalpingogram films*

Contact the radiology department of the hospital where the X-ray was performed.

Please specify that the X-ray films and the report should be sent to us for review.

□ *Operative reports*

Contact the medical records department of the hospital where the surgery was performed and ask that the medical records pertaining to the surgery be sent to us.

□ *Office notes*

Obtain all office records from physicians who have evaluated or treated you for infertility.

□ **Follow-up consultation**

After all of the tests have been completed, please set up a consultation. At that time the test results will be reviewed and a treatment plan will be developed.

INFERTILITY EVALUATION SUMMARY

Name _____ **DOB** _____

DATE	TEST	RESULT	DATE	RESULT	DATE	RESULT
☐	CD 3 FSH		☐		☐	
☐	CD 3 E2		☐		☐	
☐	CD 10 FSH (CCCT)		☐		☐	
☐	Prolactin		☐		☐	
☐	TSH		☐		☐	
☐	Thyroid antibodies		☐		☐	
☐	Testosterone					
☐	DHEA-S					
☐	17-OH-progesterone		**MALE PARTNER TESTING**			
☐	Hgb A1C		**DATE**	**TEST**	**RESULT**	
☐	Fasting insulin		☐	HIV screen		
☐	Fasting glucose		☐	Karyotype		
☐	2° glucose (GTT)		☐	Type & screen		
☐	CBC		☐	FSH		
☐	Type & screen		☐	LH		
☐	Rubella screen		☐	Testosterone		
☐	Varicella screen		☐	Prolactin		
☐	RPR		☐	Cystic fibrosis		
☐	Hepatitis screen		☐	Gaucher		
☐	HIV screen		☐	Canavan		
☐	Karyotype		☐	Tay Sachs		
☐	Lupus anticoagulant		☐	Hgb electrophoresis		
☐	Anticardiolipin ab		☐			
☐	Cystic fibrosis		☐			
☐	Gaucher					
☐	Canavan		**SEMEN ANALYSIS**			
☐	Tay Sachs		**DATE**	**Count**	**Motility**	**Morphology**
☐	Hgb electrophoresis		☐			
☐	Pap smear		☐			
☐	Mammogram		☐			
☐						
☐						

DATE	TEST	FINDINGS/COMMENTS
☐	HSG	
☐	Sono-HSG	
☐	Laparoscopy	
☐	Hysteroscopy	
☐	Endometrial Bx	

4.

Algorithms for clinical presentation

This chapter contains clinical algorithms which will aid the physician in the day to day management of the infertile couple. Each infertile couple presents with a different set of circumstances and the scope of the testing and recommended treatment will vary accordingly. It must be realized that the clinical algorithms are general guidelines regarding patient care and other circumstances, including patient choice, may dictate another course of management other than that presented.

The following clinical algorithms are presented:

Infertility evaluation

Normal evaluation

Reduced ovarian reserve

Ovulatory dysfunction

Uterine factor

Tubal/peritoneal factor

Male factor

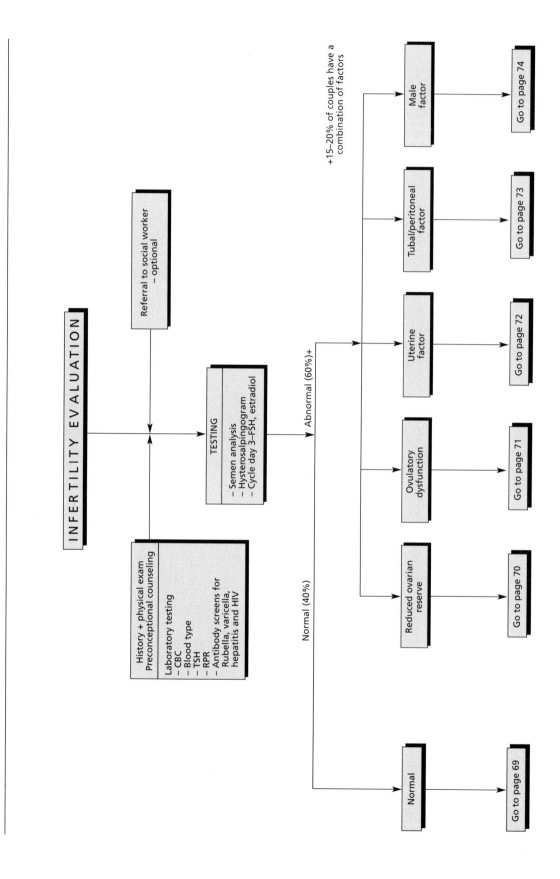

INFERTILITY EVALUATION

INFERTILITY EVALUATION

Referral to social worker – optional

History + physical exam
Preconceptional counseling

Laboratory testing
– CBC
– Blood type
– TSH
– RPR
– Antibody screens for Rubella, varicella, hepatitis and HIV

TESTING
– Semen analysis
– Hysterosalpingogram
– Cycle day 3–FSH, estradiol

Normal (40%)

Abnormal (60%)+

+15–20% of couples have a combination of factors

Normal

Go to page 69

Reduced ovarian reserve

Go to page 70

Ovulatory dysfunction

Go to page 71

Uterine factor

Go to page 72

Tubal/peritoneal factor

Go to page 73

Male factor

Go to page 74

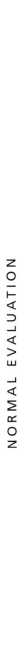

NORMAL EVALUATION

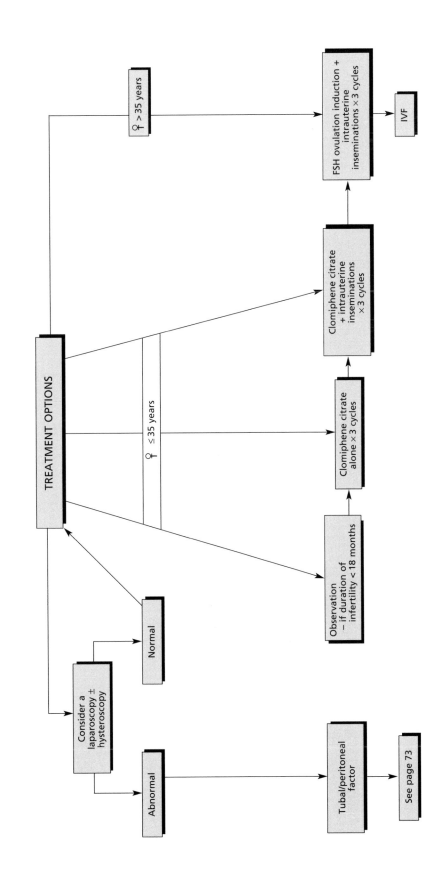

REDUCED OVARIAN RESERVE

DIAGNOSIS:

The diagnosis of reduced ovarian reserve is supported by any of the following:

1. Cycle day 3 FSH > 10 mIU/ml or estradiol > 70 pg/ml

2. Abnormal clomiphene challenge test

To perform:

- Cycle day 3 FSH, estradiol levels
- Clomiphene citrate 100 mg cycle days 5–9
- Cycle day 10 FSH level

If any of the FSH levels are > 10 mIU/ml or the estradiol is > 70 pg/ml the test is considered abnormal

3. Documented poor response to aggressive ovulation induction

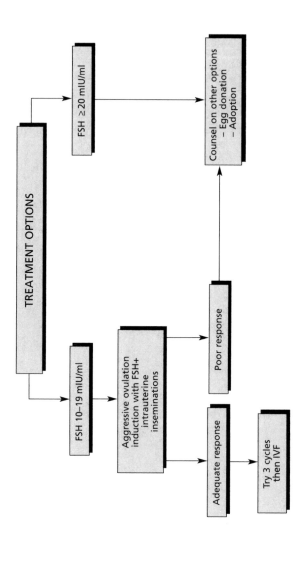

OVULATORY DYSFUNCTION

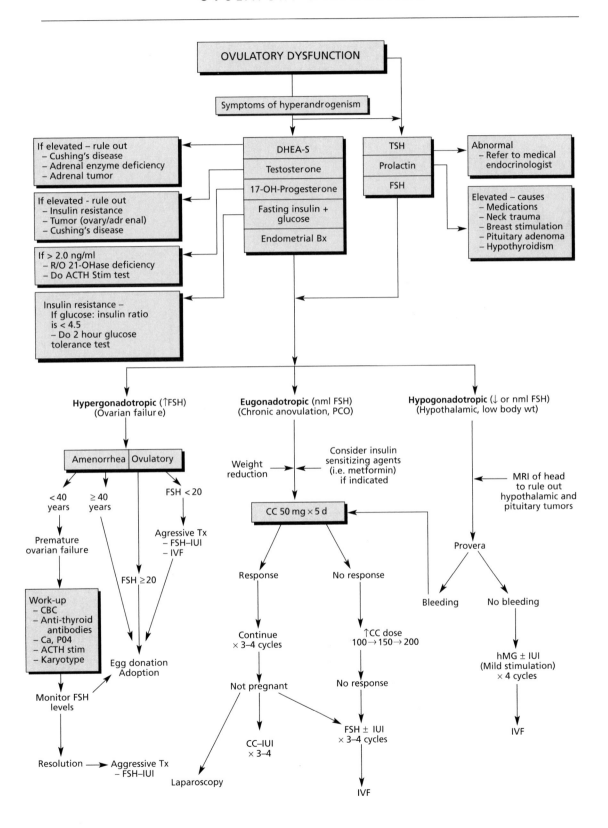

UTERINE FACTOR

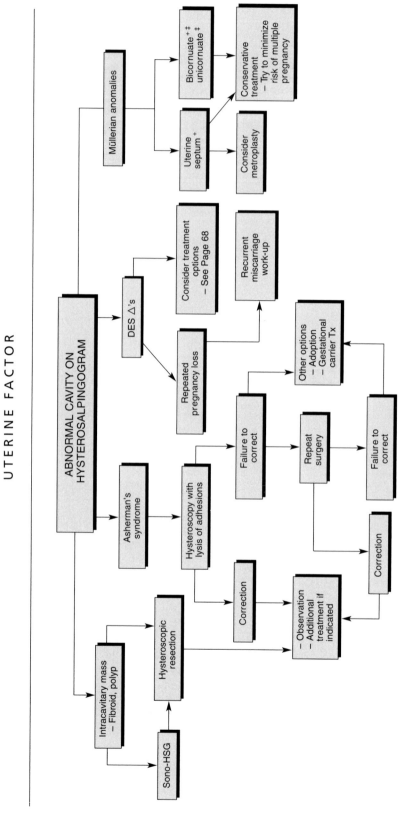

+ A laparoscopy, vaginal ultrasound, and/or MRI will help to differentiate between a uterine septum and a bicornuate uterus

‡ Renal ultrasound to rule out anomalies in cases of unicornuate or bicornuate

ABNORMAL CAVITY ON HYSTEROSALPINGOGRAM

Intracavitary mass
– Fibroid, polyp

Sono-HSG

Hysteroscopic resection

Correction

– Observation
– Additional treatment if indicated

Correction

Asherman's syndrome

Hysteroscopy with lysis of adhesions

Failure to correct

Repeat surgery

Failure to correct

Other options
– Adoption
– Gestational carrier Tx

DES Δ's

Consider treatment options
– See Page 68

Repeated pregnancy loss

Recurrent miscarriage work-up

Müllerian anomalies

Bicornuate +‡
unicornuate ‡

Uterine septum +

Conservative treatment
– Try to minimize risk of multiple pregnancy

Consider metroplasty

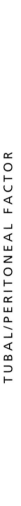

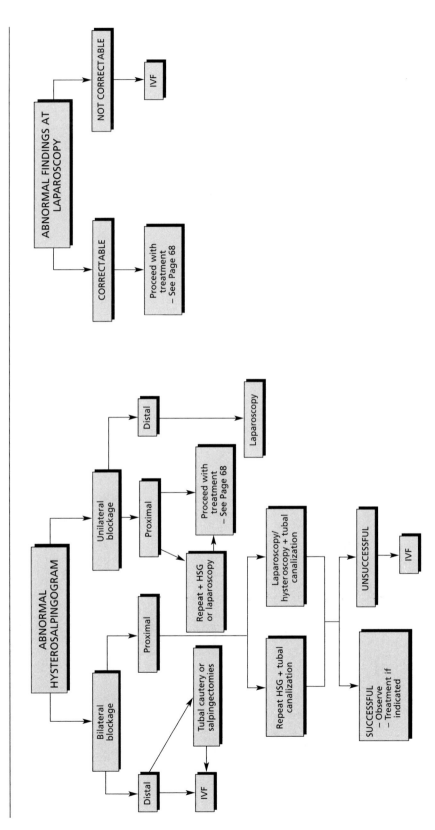

TUBAL/PERITONEAL FACTOR

ABNORMAL FINDINGS AT LAPAROSCOPY
- NOT CORRECTABLE → IVF
- CORRECTABLE → Proceed with treatment – See Page 68

ABNORMAL HYSTEROSALPINGOGRAM
- Unilateral blockage
  - Distal → Laparoscopy
  - Proximal → Proceed with treatment – See Page 68
  - Repeat + HSG or laparoscopy
- Bilateral blockage
  - Proximal
  - Distal → IVF
  - Tubal cautery or salpingectomies → IVF
- Laparoscopy/hysteroscopy + tubal canalization
- Repeat HSG + tubal canalization
- UNSUCCESSFUL → IVF
- SUCCESSFUL – Observe – Treatment if indicated

MALE FACTOR

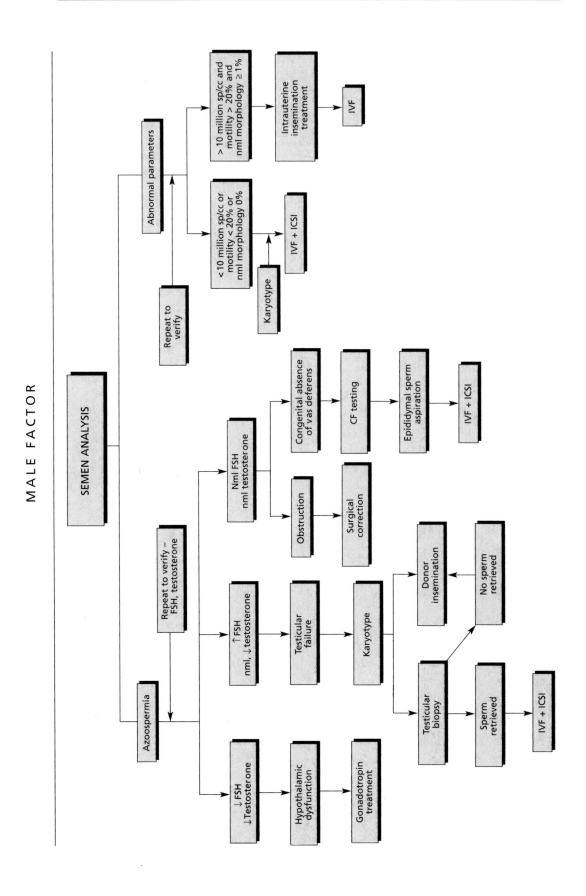

5.

Infertility treatment options: the basics

There is a spectrum of infertility treatments available for the couple and clinician to choose from. The optimal treatment is one that provides an acceptable success rate, is associated with minimal risk and is cost-effective. Taking all of these factors into consideration, the indicated treatment in cases of ovulatory dysfunction may be simple treatment with clomiphene citrate alone, while in cases of severe male factor more aggressive treatment with *in vitro* fertilization and the ICSI procedure may be indicated. In this chapter, we present the spectrum of treatment options which are available including ovulation induction, intrauterine insemination treatment, and IVF and IVF-related procedures. Medications are an integral part of these infertility treatments and are listed below. Success rates for the various treatments are discussed in Chapter 6.

OVULATION INDUCTION

Indications

Ovulation induction treatment alone is the indicated therapy for women with ovulatory dysfunction secondary to chronic anovulation or hypothalamic dysfunction. Ovulatory dysfunction that is secondary to ovarian failure is not generally corrected with the use of ovulation induction medications.

Clinical strategy

Initially, the goal is to correct the ovulatory dysfunction with clomiphene citrate (CC) because it is easy to administer, inexpensive and associated with a lower chance of a multiple pregnancy when compared to gonadotropins. If increased doses of clomiphene citrate fail to correct the ovulatory problem then treatment with gonadotropins is indicated. Typically, women with hypothalamic dysfunction do not respond to CC but do respond to human menopausal gonadotropins.

Monitoring

Patients who take CC require minimal monitoring, if any at all. Timing of intercourse can be facilitated with the use of an ovulation predictor kit. For patients receiving gonadotropins closer monitoring is required with serum estradiol testing and vaginal ultrasound examinations to measure the size of the follicles. When using gonadotropins to correct ovulatory dysfunction the goal is to get 1–2 follicles to maturity (≥ 17 mm). If too many follicles develop it may be best to cancel the cycle to prevent a multiple pregnancy and ovarian hyperstimulation.

Success rates

These are discussed in Chapter 6.

INTRAUTERINE INSEMINATION (IUI) TREATMENT WITH OVARIAN STIMULATION

Indications

This treatment may be considered in cases of unexplained infertility, cervical factor and in cases of a mild male factor.

Clinical strategy

IUI treatment involves several steps including ovarian stimulation, sperm preparation and performance of the IUI.

Ovarian stimulation

Medications are used to increase the number of eggs that are released at the time of ovulation. If the woman is under the age of 35, the ovulation induction agent of choice is CC, which is administered at a dose of 100 mg daily between cycle days 3 and 7. Testing of daily urine samples with an ovulation predictor kit is begun on cycle day 11. When the LH surge is detected by the urine testing, the insemination treatment is scheduled for the following day. For women over the age of 35 or those who have failed to achieve pregnancy after three cycles of CC-IUI, the ovulation induction agent of choice is an injectable gonadotropin (e.g. Gonal F®, Follistim®), which is started on cycle day 3. Monitoring is accomplished with vaginal ultrasound examinations and serum estradiol measurements. When adequate follicular development has resulted, ovulation is induced with human chorionic gonadotropin (hCG) and the IUI treatment is then scheduled during the peri-ovulatory period. A non-medicated approach to

FERTILITY MEDICATIONS

Clomiphene citrate (Serophene®, Clomid®): Clomiphene citrate is an oral agent that acts as a weak estrogen agonist and results in increased secretion of gonadotropins. Its primary indication is the correction of ovulatory dysfunction. This medication is described in greater detail in Chapter 7.

Gonadotropins: Gonadotropins are injectable medications used for ovulation induction for intrauterine insemination and IVF treatment. Two types of gonadotropins can be administered and are discussed below:

1. **FSH (Gonal-F®, Follistim®, Fertinex®)** – These medications contain only FSH and are administered by subcutaneous injection. These are the most commonly prescribed medications for ovulation induction.

2. **Human menopausal gonadotropins (Pergonal®, Humegon®, Repronex®)** – These medications contain equal amounts of FSH and LH, and are administered on a daily basis by intramuscular injections.

GnRH agonist (Lupron®): This is a synthetic hormone that is administered by subcutaneous injection. The administration of a GnRH agonist initially causes release of FSH and LH from the pituitary gland. However, with continued administration there is a temporary depletion of FSH and LH, which prevents a LH surge. GnRH agonists are administered with gonadotropins in women undergoing IVF treatment. The main benefit is that pretreatment with a GnRH agonist prevents a LH surge.

GnRH antagonists (Antagon™, Cetrotide™): GnRH antagonists are new medications that have become available. They reversibly bind to GnRH receptors and prevent release of FSH and LH. The major benefit of the use of GnRH antagonists in conjunction with FSH is the suppression of the LH surge. This is of great benefit for patients undergoing IVF treatment.

Human chorionic gonadotropin [hCG] (Profasi®, Pregnyl®, Ovidrel®, Novarel®): This medication contains pregnancy hormone, hCG, which functions similarly to LH. LH is an important hormone that helps to mature the eggs to allow them to become fertilized and stimulates ovulation. The administration of hCG is necessary in women who are undergoing IUI (when gonadotropins are used) and during IVF treatment.

Progesterone supplements: Progesterone supplements are used in women undergoing IVF treatment to help prepare the endometrium for implantation and support a pregnancy. Progesterone can be administered by intramuscular injection, vaginally and orally. If pregnancy occurs, the progesterone may be continued until the 10th week of pregnancy. Progesterone supplements are *not* FDA-approved for IVF treatment. However, the progesterone present in the supplements is the natural hormone and studies have confirmed there is no increased risk of congenital anomalies or health risks to women who take natural progesterone supplements during pregnancy. Refer to Chapter 8 for a more detailed discussion about the role of progesterone supplementation.

IUI treatment is an option but should be discouraged because of the low success rate.

Preparation of the semen sample

Inseminations are generally performed on 1 or 2 consecutive days around the time of ovulation. On the days of the IUI treatments, the male partner will be asked to produce a semen sample. It is preferable that the semen sample is produced on site, but it can be produced at home and then transported to the laboratory. The sperm concentration and motility of the semen sample are assessed. The semen sample is then washed and prepared.

Intrauterine inseminations

To perform the IUI treatments a speculum examination is performed and the cervix is visualized. The washed sperm sample is loaded into a catheter, which is inserted through the cervical canal and into the uterine cavity. Following the inseminations, normal activity can be resumed and a pregnancy test is scheduled 14 days later.

Success rates

These are discussed in Chapter 6.

IVF AND RELATED PROCEDURES

Introduction

The assisted reproductive technologies (ART) are advanced treatments that can be used when conventional treatment has failed, the Fallopian tubes are damaged or a severe male factor is present. IVF, the first ART procedure, was introduced over 20 years ago. Since then other ART procedures have been developed which are variations of the IVF procedure. This section will provide a basic understanding of the various ART procedures and the laboratory techniques that can be used.

IVF

IVF is the most commonly performed ART procedure and accounts for over 95% of ART cases performed in this country. The treatment was originally introduced for tubal factor infertility but it can be utilized for any type of infertility that is not corrected with conventional treatment. IVF is also the indicated treatment in cases of severe male factor. IVF treatment consists of several steps, which are discussed below.

Ovarian stimulation

During a natural cycle, only one mature ovarian follicle develops which results in the ovulation of a single egg. The goal of ovulation induction is to use medications to stimulate the growth of multiple ovarian follicles to a stage of maturity. The success rate following IVF is directly related to the number of oocytes that are retrieved and the number of embryos that are transferred. The ovulation induction protocols that we use are described below.

Pituitary down-regulation with a GnRH agonist   This is the ovarian stimulation protocol that is used by most IVF programs. It involves daily injections of a GnRH agonist, Lupron®, which is administered until 'down-regulation' of pituitary GnRH receptors has occurred and pituitary FSH and LH release is reduced to a minimum. Generally, the GnRH agonist has to be administered for a period of 10–15 days before down-regulation has occurred which is confirmed by the onset of menses and a serum estradiol level that is less than 50 pg/ml. The quickest way to achieve down-regulation is to start the GnRH agonist in the mid-luteal phase. It can also be started in the early follicular phase with the onset of menses. The major advantage of the down-regulation protocol is that there is suppression of the LH surge. After down-regulation has occurred the dose of the GnRH agonist is reduced and the ovulation induction is initiated with daily FSH injections.

Microdose-Lupron protocol   This protocol is used for women who are poor responders or who have evidence of reduced ovarian reserve. This protocol involves the administration of oral contraceptives for a period of 3 weeks. Theoretically, the administration of the oral contraceptive puts the ovaries to rest. After the 3-week course of the oral contraceptives has been completed, then microdoses of Lupron and FSH are administered twice daily. When Lupron is administered in this fashion it acts as a stimulatory agent because it induces the release of FSH and LH. In addition, there is inhibition of the LH surge.

Pituitary suppression with a GnRH antagonist   Another protocol that is used utilizes a GnRH antagonist, which suppresses a LH surge. In contrast to the GnRH agonist, the pituitary suppression achieved by the GnRH antagonist is more rapid. For this protocol, gonadotropins are initiated on cycle day 2. When the lead follicle reaches a diameter of 14 mm the GnRH antagonist is administered (with the gonadotropins) on a daily basis.

Monitoring   During the ovarian stimulation, the woman's response to treatment is monitored with serum estradiol levels and vaginal ultrasound examinations. The goal of the ovulation induction is to develop at least three mature follicles. A mature follicle is one that is at least 15–17 mm in diameter. Once this is achieved the FSH and other medications are discontinued. The woman then takes a single injection of hCG, which further matures the eggs to allow them to become fertilized. If it is judged that the response is insufficient the cycle is cancelled and the treatment plan is reassessed.

Egg retrieval

The egg retrieval is performed under vaginal ultrasound guidance. After the vaginal ultrasound is placed in the vagina and the ovarian follicles are located, a needle is directed through the back wall of the vagina and directly into the ovarian follicles (Figure 5.1). The fluid is aspirated and then examined by an embryologist to see if an egg has been retrieved (Figure 5.2). All follicles within both ovaries are aspirated. Once the eggs are retrieved they are placed in culture plates with nutrient media and then placed in the incubator. The procedure is performed under a light anesthesia and takes less than 5–10 minutes to perform. Progesterone is started the evening after the egg retrieval.

Sperm insemination

On the day of egg retrieval, a sperm sample is obtained and prepared to select out the most motile sperm. The motile sperm are placed next to the eggs in a culture dish, which is then placed in the incubator. The following morning, the eggs are examined to determine whether fertilization has occurred. A fertilized egg is shown in Figure 5.3. Note the two pronucleii (one from the sperm and the other from the egg) present within the egg. Within a few hours the nucleii unite and the embryo will start to divide (Figure 5.4).

Embryo transfer

If fertilization has resulted, then the embryo transfer is performed usually 72 hours after the egg retrieval. Generally, two to five embryos are transferred into the uterine cavity. At this stage, good quality embryos are usually between 6–10 cells in development. The recommended number of embryos to transfer can be influenced by the woman's age, cause of the infertility, previous pregnancy history and other factors. Extra embryos that are of sufficient quality

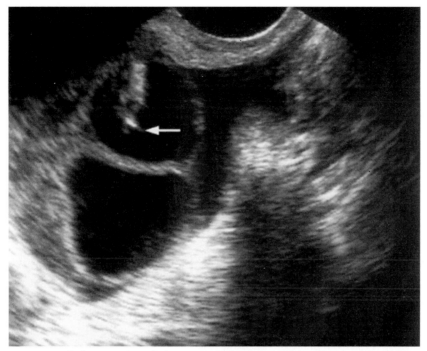

Figure 5.1 Vaginal ultrasound-guided egg retrieval. This is an ultrasound image taken at the time of an egg retrieval. During the procedure the ovary is positioned on the other side of the vaginal wall. A needle has been inserted through the vaginal wall and the tip of the needle is positioned in the center of the follicle (see arrow). After proper placement of the needle the fluid from the follicle is aspirated

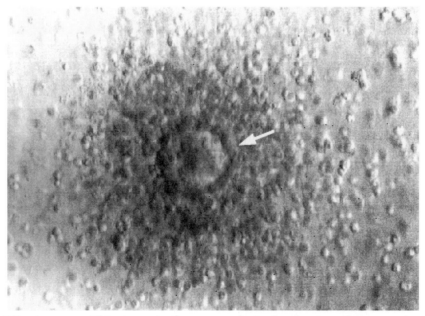

Figure 5.2 An oocyte. This picture is of an oocyte obtained at the time of an egg retrieval. The oocyte (see arrow) is surrounded by a group of granulosa cells called the cumulus. During normal fertilization the acrosome of the sperm releases enzymes which disperse the cumulus cells therefore allowing the sperm to penetrate and fertilize the oocyte

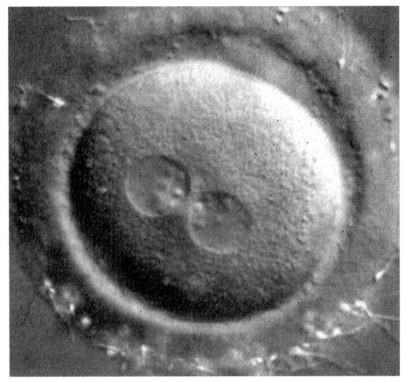

Figure 5.3 A fertilized egg. Note the two pronuclei (one from the sperm and one from the egg) present within the egg

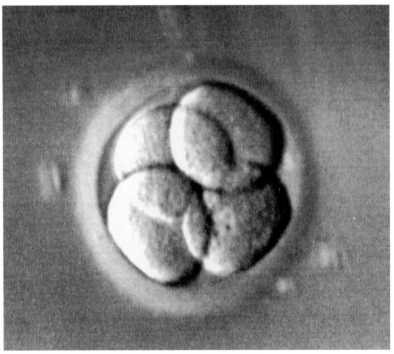

Figure 5.4 A four-cell embryo. This stage of development is achieved at 24–48 hours after fertilization. Note the outer membrane called the zona pellucida that surrounds the embryo

can be frozen and stored for future use. A serum pregnancy test is conducted 11 days later.

Success rates

These are discussed in Chapter 6.

IVF-related procedures

Frozen embryo transfer (FET)

Embryos that are cryopreserved during an IVF or GIFT procedure can be replaced after a spontaneous ovulation or the creation of an 'artificial' endometrium with oral estrogen and progesterone. The success rate following this procedure is between 10 and 20% and is dependent on the number and quality of embryos that are transferred. The main advantage of a frozen embryo transfer as compared to a medicated IVF cycle is that ovulation induction drugs are not taken and, obviously, an egg retrieval is not performed. It is reassuring that there is no increased risk of congenital anomalies in infants born following the transfer of cryopreserved embryos.

Natural cycle IVF

For couples who want to minimize the risk of a multiple pregnancy or would like to avoid the risks of the ovulation induction drugs, a natural cycle IVF approach can be considered. The woman undergoes monitoring with blood work and ultrasound examinations beginning on cycle day 10. The hCG is administered when a mature follicle is identified. If a LH surge occurs then the cycle is cancelled. The goal of the natural cycle approach is the retrieval of one egg and the replacement of one embryo. The success rate is less than 5% which is a major disadvantage of this approach.

Gamete intrafallopian transfer (GIFT)

This treatment involves the first two steps of IVF treatment: ovulation induction and egg retrieval. In contrast to IVF, the GIFT procedure places the eggs and sperm in the Fallopian tube, allowing the tube to be the natural incubator. Usually, four to six eggs are replaced and all remaining eggs can be fertilized by the standard IVF technique and then the embryos are frozen. The disadvantage of the GIFT procedure is that a laparoscopy has to be performed under general anesthesia. A prerequisite to performing the GIFT procedure is that the woman must have at least one normal Fallopian tube. This procedure was quite popular in years past but as the IVF pregnancy rates have continued to increase there are fewer reasons to perform this procedure. Actually less than 2% of ART procedures are GIFT. Indications for resorting to GIFT instead of IVF include altered cervical anatomy that prevents a successful uterine transfer and for religious reasons.

Tubal embryo transfer (TET)

This treatment involves the first three steps of IVF: ovulation induction, egg retrieval and fertilization of the eggs in the laboratory. In contrast to IVF, the TET procedure involves the laparoscopic placement of the embryos in the Fallopian tube(s), allowing the tube to be the natural incubator. Usually, two to four embryos are replaced. The disadvantage of the TET procedure is that two separate procedures are performed requiring anesthesia including the egg retrieval and a laparoscopy. This procedure is rarely performed but might be considered when there is altered cervical anatomy and the GIFT procedure is not an option (i.e. when the ICSI procedure is required).

Egg donation

Egg donation can be considered for a woman who is a poor responder to the ovulation induction medications, has evidence of reduced ovarian reserve or is a carrier of a genetic condition. All of the steps of IVF are performed except the egg donor undergoes the ovulation induction and egg retrieval. Once the eggs are retrieved, they are then fertilized with the recipient's husband's sperm. The recipient is treated with hormones including estrogen and progesterone, which create an endometrium that will allow implantation of the embryos. The donor can be anonymous or known (i.e. a relative, friend). Before this treatment is begun all parties involved should undergo medical, psychological and legal counseling.

Gestational carrier treatment

The existence of the embryos outside of the woman's body creates the possibility of placement of the embryos into a second woman (gestational carrier) who then carries the pregnancy. The intention following the delivery is to unite the baby or babies with the couple who will be the rearing parents. Indications for gestational carrier treatment are when the woman has no uterus, a congenitally deformed uterus, a uterus which is unable to support a pregnancy, or has a medical condition which precludes her from successfully carrying a pregnancy. All the steps of IVF treatment are performed except the embryos are transferred into a gestational carrier. Before this treatment is begun, all parties involved must undergo medical, psychological and legal counseling.

Embryo donation

When a couple decides that they do not want any more children or stop treatment they are forced to make difficult decisions regarding their frozen embryos. Because of religious or moral beliefs, some couples find it unacceptable to discard the embryos. One option is to donate the embryos to another couple. Embryo donation is just emerging as a treatment option for infertile couples and will be used more and more in the future. Embryo donation is very similar to an adoption. Medical, psychological and legal counseling are important components of the treatment.

Epididymal sperm aspiration

In some cases of azoospermia, the sperm are being produced but do not find their way to the ejaculate. This may be the result of an obstruction (e.g. previous vasectomy, infection), congenital absence of the vas deferens or in cases of severely impaired sperm production. In these cases, aspiration of epididymal sperm or testicular sperm by a urologist may be considered. In years past, the only way to aspirate epididymal sperm was via the microscopic epididymal sperm aspiration (MESA) procedure. This procedure is performed in the operating room under general anesthesia. More recently, the percutaneous epididymal sperm aspiration (PESA) procedure has become more popular. It can be accomplished under local anesthesia and a much shorter recuperation than the MESA procedure. If epididymal sperm aspiration does not produce viable sperm the urologist can resort to the testicular sperm extraction (TESE). In all cases of sperm aspiration, the motility of the samples is quite poor so the ICSI procedure must be performed. To accomplish this procedure there must be coordination with the urologist and the IVF team. The sperm aspiration can be performed on the day of the oocyte recovery or prior to the IVF cycle and the samples frozen.

Laboratory procedures

Standard IVF culture

The eggs and sperm are cultured in a small volume of culture medium under oil. This is the standard technique that is used in cases in which there is no contributory male factor. Generally, 8000–12 000 motile sperm are added to the microdrops containing the eggs.

Intracytoplasmic sperm injection (ICSI)

This is a technique that involves the injection of a single sperm directly into the oocyte (Figure 5.5). This procedure has been used in couples who have no fertilization following a previous IVF cycle or in cases of a severe male factor. Fertilization rates following this procedure are between 50 and 70%. Males with severe oligospermia (count < 5 million sperm/cc) are at greater risk for being a carrier of cystic fibrosis and having a chromosomal abnormality. Therefore, they should have a cystic fibrosis screen and a karyotype performed. Couples should be counseled that there is an increased risk of sex chromosomal anomalies in infants born following the ICSI procedure. The rate of sex chromosomal aneuploidy in the general population is 0.2% and 0.8% following the ICSI procedure. Couples may opt for a genetic amniocentesis after pregnancy is established. Studies have confirmed that some cases of male factor infertility are caused by microdeletions on the Y chromosome. Couples should be counseled that this genetic defect could be transmitted to an offspring.

Assisted hatching

Assisted hatching is a procedure in which the zona pellucida, the outer membrane surrounding the embryo, is thinned by the application of a dilute acidic

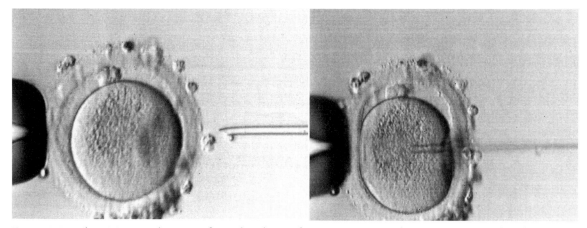

Figure 5.5 The ICSI procedure is performed with very fine instruments under a microscope. After the granulosa cells have been stripped away from the oocyte with enzymes, the oocyte is held in place by a holding pipette. The other pipette which is much smaller and sharper is used to pick up a single sperm. The smaller pipette is then brought into proper position (left panel) and then inserted through the zona pellucida and into the cytoplasm of the oocyte where the sperm is injected (right panel)

solution and mechanically disrupted. Studies have suggested that, in certain women, the zona pellucida may undergo a hardening process. This may interfere with embryo hatching which is a necessary step for implantation. However, the published studies are inconclusive about the benefit of this procedure. We do not feel that it should be performed routinely but may be considered in cases of advanced maternal age or failure to achieve a pregnancy after multiple IVF cycles.

Blastocyst culture

The blastocyst stage of embryonic development occurs just prior to implantation. The blastocyst is an embryo made up of 50–100 cells and reaches this stage of development 5–6 days after the egg retrieval (Figure 5.6). During IVF treatment, the standard timing of the embryo transfer has been 3 days after the egg retrieval. At this stage, the embryos are between 5 and 10 cells in development. Until recently, we did not have the ability to culture embryos past this stage. Over the past few years commercially available culture media have become available and will support more advanced embryonic growth to the blastocyst stage in the laboratory. Generally, 30–50% of embryos develop to the blastocyst stage. Therefore, the benefit from blastocyst culture is that it allows the selection of the best quality embryos. Further, by reducing the number of blastocysts that are transferred to two, the chance of a high-order multiple pregnancy is significantly reduced and the patient has an excellent chance of

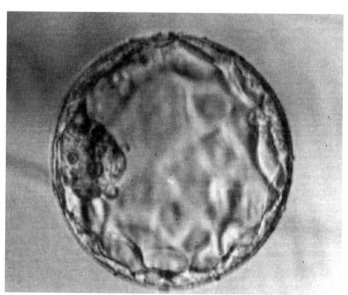

Figure 5.6 A blastocyst. Approximately 30–50% of embryos will develop to the blastocyst state 5–6 days after the egg retrieval. The blastocyst is made up of over 50–100 cells

pregnancy. In our experience with the transfer of two blastocysts there is, approximately, a 40% chance of pregnancy; if pregnancy is established there is a 30% chance of a multiple pregnancy.

Preimplantation genetic diagnosis (PGD)

In the past when a couple was at risk of having a child with a genetic condition, the only options for genetic diagnosis were a chorionic villous sampling or a genetic amniocentesis. These choices are not optimal because terminating a pregnancy can be quite stressful and for many couples pregnancy termination is not considered an option. PGD provides couples with another option. The refinement of micromanipulation techniques in the IVF laboratory has provided the ability to perform genetic diagnosis on a single blastomere that is removed from the embryo prior to transfer. The first successful case of PGD was performed in 1990 for a couple who were at risk of having a child with cystic fibrosis. Since that time other centers world-wide have developed the expertise to perform PGD. PGD can be performed for autosomal recessive and dominant conditions, to assess aneuploidy and for translocations. PGD is an emerging technology and as more and more genetic probes become available there will be an increased demand for this procedure.

6.

Success rates of infertility treatment: what to tell your patients

In order to counsel infertile couples the clinician must have an understanding of success rates for the various treatments. In other areas of medicine, when a patient undergoes treatment for a medical problem, a cure rate of 80–90% or even 100% is expected. Unfortunately, this is not true when treating infertility. The explanation is simple – *the human reproductive system is inefficient*. It is important that this fact is conveyed to our patients. In optimal circumstances, a normal fertile couple in the general population has only a 15–20% chance of achieving a pregnancy during any menstrual cycle. Further, if pregnancy is established, there is a 20–30% chance of a pregnancy loss. Taking these statistics into consideration, we often wonder how any couple is able to achieve a successful pregnancy. While the overall chance of pregnancy during any one cycle in optimal circumstances is low, the cumulative pregnancy rate over time continues to go up. This is true for the normal fertile couple in the general population and the infertile couple undergoing treatment. In this Chapter, we discuss factors that affect treatment outcome and present success rates for the various infertility treatments.

FACTORS AFFECTING TREATMENT OUTCOME

The goal of infertility treatment is to create the optimal conditions for a conception. A variety of treatments are available which have varying success rates. The success of any treatment is influenced by known and unknown factors. Some of these factors are discussed below.

Maternal age

One of the most important factors that influences a couple's fertility is the woman's age. Generally, younger women have a greater quantity and quality of eggs that once fertilized are more likely to implant in the uterus and result in a pregnancy. Further, the chance of a miscarriage is lower in younger women. The decreased fertility associated with advancing age is a gradual process that seems to begin around age 25 and then accelerates after the age of 40. For this reason, women over the age of 40 should be counseled about the decreased chances of pregnancy even with aggressive treatment, such as *in vitro* fertilization (Figure 6.1). Treatment is contraindicated in women who are 45 years and older because of the dismal chance of a successful outcome. Some have even questioned whether treatment is justified in women who are 43 and 44 years of age. These women of advanced reproductive age should be counseled and encouraged to pursue other more fruitful options such as egg donation and adoption.

Ovarian reserve

A measurement of cycle day 3 FSH and estradiol levels helps to assess the degree of ovarian reserve. If either the FSH or estradiol level is elevated, reduced ovarian reserve should be suspected. Reduced ovarian reserve is associated with a reduced chance of pregnancy and a higher chance of miscarriage[18]. This information helps the clinician in counseling the couple on treatment options. However, there are limitations in the correlation between the FSH levels and fertility. In our experience, we have identified some women who have elevated FSH levels but normal fertility. We have also observed that other women

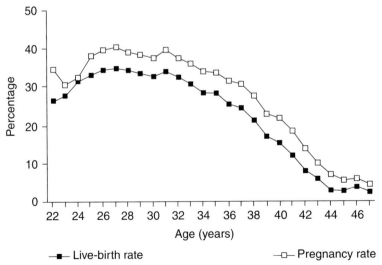

Figure 6.1   Pregnancy and live-birth rates for ART cycles using fresh (non-donor) embryos by age of the woman. Obtained from published data from the National Centers for Disease Control Report, *1998 Assisted Reproductive Technology Success Rates*

have fluctuations in their FSH levels from cycle to cycle and over a period of time. However, even a single abnormal level is associated with a reduced prognosis.

Semen quality

The semen analysis is the best test we have to evaluate a male's fertility potential. However, the semen analysis does have its limitations since it is only a quantitative assessment of the semen sample and absolute thresholds for the semen parameters have not been determined that truly differentiate between fertile and infertile males. The degree of the male factor may influence the chances of pregnancy either spontaneously or with conservative treatment (i.e. intrauterine inseminations). Since the introduction of intracytoplasmic sperm injection (ICSI) in 1994, the severity of the male factor is less important with IVF treatment. With the ICSI procedure, all that is needed is a single viable sperm for each oocyte that is inseminated. Fertilization rates following the ICSI procedure are between 50 and 70%. It is of interest that embryos resulting from the ICSI procedure and standard insemination have the same chances of implantation.

Cause of the infertility

Women with ovulatory problems, except those with reduced ovarian reserve, tend to have higher pregnancy rates with the various treatments. Women with tubal factor infertility or severe male factor infertility seem to fair poorly with conservative interventions (i.e. ovulation induction with or without intra-uterine inseminations). While the cause of the infertility may impact on success rates of the conservative treatments there is virtually little difference between the success rates for the different diagnostic categories with IVF treatment (Figure 6.2).

Duration of the infertility

From a theoretical standpoint it seems logical that a couple with a longer duration of infertility would experience a lower chance of success following treatment. However, published data do not support this contention[52]. There-fore, couples with long-standing infertility of 10 or more years should not be discouraged from undergoing treatment.

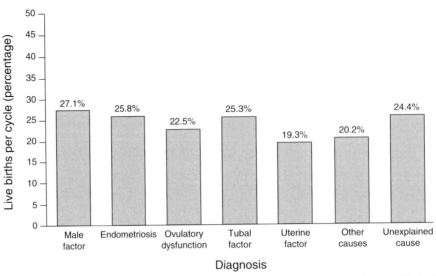

Figure 6.2 Live-birth rates following ART by primary diagnosis. Obtained from published data from the National Centers for Disease Control Report, *1998 Assisted Reproductive Technology Success Rates*

Pregnancy history

The success of the infertility treatment is influenced by the prior pregnancy history. Women who have had a successful pregnancy have a greater chance of success when undergoing infertility treatment. More specifically for those pursing IVF treatment, women with a prior live born have a 15–20% greater chance of success[53].

Toxic exposures

Women who smoke have half the chance of achieving pregnancy compared to non-smokers[9,10]. Other lifestyle issues that have been shown to reduce the chances of pregnancy include the use of caffeine and alcohol[8,13]. Environmental exposures can also be of detriment (see Chapter 2).

SUCCESS RATES FOLLOWING CONSERVATIVE TREATMENT

The average success rates for the various conservative treatment options are shown in Table 6.1. It must be realized that these are averages for populations and any individual couple may have a higher or lower success rate depending on their circumstances. For instance, women with ovulatory dysfunction tend to have higher success rates and a higher chance of a multiple pregnancy. Women who have advanced age (> 40 years), a tubal/peritoneal factor or have a

Table 6.1 Success rates for conservative infertility treatment options

Treatment	Success rate (per cycle) (%)	Multiple pregnancy rate (%)
Observation	3–4	1
Non-medicated IUI	4	1
Clomiphene citrate	6	10
Clomiphene citrate–IUI	8–10	10
FSH	10	15–20
FSH–IUI	15–18	20–25

IUI, intrauterine insemination; FSH, follicle stimulating hormone injections

contributory male factor have lower success rates following these conservative treatments.

SUCCESS RATES FOLLOWING TREATMENT WITH IVF AND RELATED PROCEDURES

IVF was the first reproductive technology that was introduced over 20 years ago. After it was first introduced, it was viewed as an investigational procedure but now IVF treatment is a standard treatment for the infertile couple. It was originally developed to treat tubal factor infertility but now it is a treatment that can be considered for any cause of infertility that fails to respond to conservative treatment. Over the years, IVF success rates have continued to rise (Figure 6.3). The explanation for the increased success rate is many fold, including improved ovulation induction medications, refined laboratory techniques and the introduction of the intracytoplasmic sperm injection (ICSI) procedure.

Gamete intrafallopian transfer (GIFT) was introduced in the mid-1980s and was offered as an alternative to IVF. Initially, after it was introduced, the success rate following a GIFT procedure was higher than IVF, but, with refinements in IVF treatment, this trend has been reversed. Therefore, the indications for doing the GIFT procedure have decreased. Presently, the two major indications for the performance of GIFT are for religious reasons or the inability of passing a catheter through a difficult cervix into the uterine cavity. Furthermore, the GIFT procedure is more risky than IVF since it is more invasive and has to be performed under general anesthesia. All of these factors have resulted in a dramatic decrease in the performance of the procedure. In the United States, the percentage of ART cases that were GIFT peaked at 21% in 1989 and was only 2% in 1998.

Since passage of the Fertility Clinic Success Rate and Certification Act of 1992 it is mandatory that all IVF centers in the United States submit their annual success rates to a federal registry. Currently, this is a joint venture of the

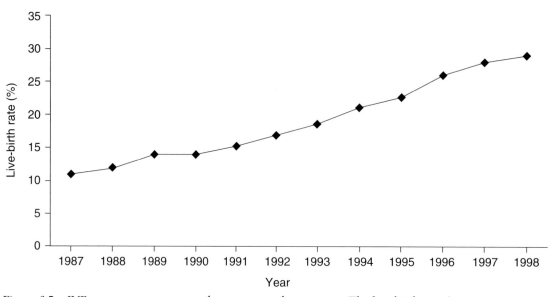

Figure 6.3 IVF treatment success rates have continued to increase. The live-birth rate (per oocyte retrieval) has increased 2.5 fold between 1987 and 1998. Data were obtained from the Society of the Assisted Reproductive Technologies (SART) registry statistics that are published on an annual basis. The increase in the success rates has been paralleled by an increased number of ART procedures that have been performed in the United States. In 1987, a total of 8725 retrievals were performed and, in 1998, a total of 53 154 procedures were carried out

United States Centers for Disease Control (CDC) and the Society of the Assisted Reproductive Technologies (SART), a subsidiary of the American Society for Reproductive Medicine (ASRM). After the annual data have been compiled, a finalized report is published and made available to the public for review. The published document includes a summary of national and clinic-specific success rates. The main impetus behind this law is that the reporting of clinic success rates would help the infertile couple select the 'best' IVF clinic for their treatment. Unfortunately, there are several shortcomings to this process. Because the published data are based on live-birth rates the most recent data that have been published are 2–3 years old and may not reflect a clinic's current success rate. Another pitfall to the interpretation of the data, is that there is no way to determine the inclusion and exclusion criteria that any individual center used in selecting patients for treatment. Therefore, as these criteria are highly variable for each program, center-by-center comparison of success rates is not valid. An unfortunate outcome to the process is that some IVF centers have used the published data for marketing purposes. Despite these shortcomings, a major benefit of the data collection is to follow national trends and success rates of the various ART procedures. To help you with the counseling of your patients we are presenting the national summary of the most recent published report, *The*

Table 6.2 Live-birth rates by age group for various ART procedures. National IVF statistics

| Treatment | Live-birth rates by age group (%) | | | | |
	< 35 years	35–37 years	38–40 years	> 40 years	Multiple pregnancy rate
IVF (± ICSI)*	32	26	18	8	39[†]
Frozen embryo transfer[‡]	21	19	18	13	N/A
Egg donation[‡]	42	44	40	41	N/A

* Live-birth rates per cycle initiated
[†] percentage of multiple pregnancies includes 28% twin and 11% triplets or more
[‡] live-birth rates per embryo transfer
N/A, not available

1998 ART Success Rates Report (Table 6.2). It can also be viewed online via *www.cdc.gov/nccdphp/drh/art/htm*. A hard copy of the report can be requested by calling the CDC (1–770–488–5372).

CONCLUSION

When treating the infertile couple, the clinician can choose from a number of different treatment options. The selection of any particular treatment is not solely based on its success rate. If this was the case, every infertile couple would undergo treatment with IVF. The appropriate treatment is one that maximizes success, minimizes risk and is cost-effective. In some cases, the treatment of choice is clomiphene citrate with timed intercourse, whereas, in other cases, the indicated treatment may be IVF.

7.

Clomiphene citrate

INTRODUCTION

Clomiphene citrate was first introduced over 30 years ago and is the most commonly prescribed medication for the infertile woman. It can be prescribed for different reasons, but its primary indication is for the correction of ovulatory dysfunction. When compared to other ovulation induction agents, clomiphene citrate is inexpensive, easy to administer and does not require intense monitoring. This chapter will provide the clinician with a better understanding of this medication and its clinical applications. In addition, other medications that can be used in conjunction with clomiphene citrate will also be discussed.

PHARMACOLOGY

Clomiphene citrate is a triphenylethylene derivative that is related to tamoxifen and diethylstilbestrol. Clomiphene citrate exists in two isomeric forms, zuclomiphene and enclomiphene citrate. The pharmacological effect of this medication is from the zuclomiphene citrate isomer. The two available agents, under the trade names of Serophene® and Clomid®, contain equal amounts of these two isomers. Clomiphene citrate is a weak estrogen agonist and binds to hypothalamic estrogen receptors, which decreases the replenishment of these receptors. The hypothalamus responds to the *psuedo*-hypoestrogenic state by increasing GnRH release, which, in turn, increases the secretion of FSH and LH from the anterior pituitary. Clomiphene citrate has a half-life of 5 days and can be detected in the blood up to 6–8 weeks after administration. Despite the long half-life of clomiphene citrate, there there are no reported increases in congenital anomalies that can be attributed to the use of this medication.

DOSAGE AND ADMINISTRATION

Clomiphene citrate is available in 50 mg tablets. The initial recommended dose of clomiphene citrate is 50 mg daily for 5 days following either a spontaneous or progesterone-induced menstrual period. Traditionally, clomiphene citrate has been administered between cycle days 5 and 9; however, the 5-day therapy can be started on cycle days 3, 4 or 5. Ovulation can be monitored with a basal body temperature chart or an ovulation predictor kit. Some couples find that the monitoring adds to the anxiety and stress of the process. For this reason, couples may find it more desirable and less stressful to have intercourse every other day between cycle days 10 and 18, which should be adequate. For the anovulatory patient, if the cycles are less than 35 days then the effective dose of clomiphene citrate should be maintained for 3–4 cycles. If the cycle length is greater than 35 days then the dose can be increased in a stepwise fashion to 100 and then to 150 mg daily for 5 days until an adequate therapeutic response is evident. Although higher doses up to 200 or 250 mg per day may be attempted, the majority of pregnancies occur at dosages of 150 mg daily or less. If the patient with chronic anovulation does not respond to a dose of 150 mg daily then our approach is to proceed on with injectable gonadotropins.

RISKS AND COMPLICATIONS

Before prescribing clomiphene citrate the following issues should be discussed with the patient concerning this medication. Informed consent is part of the treatment process and should be documented in the chart. A sample informed consent that we have developed for ovulation induction appears in Chapter 10.

Side-effects

Since clomiphene citrate is a synthetic hormonal agent, side-effects are common but are not dose-related. Many of the side-effects that result are related to the *pseudo*-hypoestrogenic state that is created. The more common side-effects include: vasomotor symptoms (10%), abdominal discomfort (6%), breast discomfort (2%), nausea/vomiting (2%), visual symptoms (2%) and headaches (1%). The use of ovulation inductions agents, especially clomiphene citrate, may result in more significant pain associated with ovulation. Patients should also be made aware that the medication can cause emotional irritability. While most women are able to deal with this side-effect others find it intolerable.

Multiple pregnancy

As with any medication that stimulates the ovaries, there is always a risk of ovulation of multiple oocytes that can result in a multiple pregnancy. The chance of a multiple pregnancy in the general population following a natural conception is 1% and is 8–10% following treatment with clomiphene citrate. The majority of these multiple pregnancies are twin gestations but couples should be counseled that there is a 1% chance of a triplet pregnancy.

Ovarian hyperstimulation

A common side-effect that can occur with any ovulation induction agent is the formation of ovarian cysts following ovulation. In most cases, these cysts do not produce symptoms and resolve within a few weeks after the onset of the menses. Ovarian hyperstimulation syndrome is the result of more significant cystic enlargement of the ovaries and the accumulation of ascites. The pathogenesis of ovarian hyperstimulation is poorly understood. In addition to the abdominal distention and pain that can be experienced, the woman may also have nausea, vomiting and difficulty breathing. In severe cases, this can be a life-threatening condition, which may necessitate hospitalization. Complications occur because of third spacing of fluids into the abdominal cavity, which can result in the development of hemoconcentration. Ovarian hyperstimulation occurs rarely with clomiphene citrate and is more common with the use of the injectable gonadotropins.

Ovarian cancer risk

There has been ongoing concern about a potential risk of ovarian cancer following the use of ovulation induction[54,55]. However, a cause and effect association has not been established. Nevertheless, patients should be counseled on this potential risk.

INDICATIONS FOR CLOMIPHENE CITRATE TREATMENT

Unexplained infertility

In clinical practice, clomiphene citrate is most commonly prescribed for the woman with unexplained infertility. However, published data are inconclusive concerning the benefits of clomiphene citrate used in this circumstance[56–58]. Nevertheless, some couples and clinicians feel that this is a reasonable treatment. As with any therapy, most pregnancies are achieved within the first few months of treatment. Therefore, the duration of treatment should be limited to 3–4 months at which time the treatment plan should be reassessed.

Recommended dosage: 50–100 mg administered between cycle days 3 and 7. Limit duration of treatment to 3–4 months. Instruct couples to use an ovulation predictor kit or have intercourse every other day between cycle days 10 and 18.

Pregnancy rate: 6% per cycle

Ovulatory dysfunction

The causes of ovulatory dysfunction can be varied and can be categorized into hypergonadotropic (ovarian failure), eugonadotropic (chronic anovulation) and hypogonadotropic (hypothalamic, weight-related) states (refer to *Clinical Algorithms* in Chapter 4). Women who have ovarian failure or are perimenopausal generally do not respond to clomiphene citrate favorably. Those women with hypothalamic amenorrhea who fail to have a progesterone withdrawal bleed also respond poorly to this medication. These women are more effectively treated with low-dose injectable human menopausal gonadotropins. Patients with chronic anovulation or oligomenorrhea generally respond well to clomiphene citrate. If either thyroid or prolactin dysfunction is evident then this needs to be evaluated and corrected before proceeding with treatment. In some cases, correction of these imbalances will resolve the ovulatory dysfunction. Patients who present with hyperandrogenism should have serum androgens assessed (e.g. testosterone, 17-hydroxyprogesterone, dehydroepiandrosterone sulfate (DHEAS)) and an assessment of the glucose metabolism (a fasting insulin and glucose). Any abnormalities noted during this work-up may necessitate further evaluation.

Recommended dosage: The initial dose of clomiphene citrate is 50 mg on cycle days 3–7. If the menstrual cycle is less than 35 days, then the current dose should be continued for three cycles. Instruct couples to use an ovulation predictor kit or time intercourse around the predicted peri-ovulatory period. If the cycles are greater than 35 days, the dosage of the clomiphene citrate should be increased in a stepwise fashion to 100 mg for 5 days. If this dose is in adequate, then increase the dose to 150 mg. If pregnancy is not achieved despite three ovulatory cycles, then other factors should be ruled out. If no other factors are identified then intrauterine inseminations can be added to the clomiphene citrate treatment.

Outcome: Proceeding in the stepwise fashion as described above, the percentages of patients that ovulate on the 50 mg, 100 mg and 150 mg dosage regimens are 50%, 22% and 12%, respectively[59]. However, despite these high ovulatory rates with clomiphene citrate treatment, only 40–50% of women will achieve pregnancy[60].

Pregnancy rate: 10% per ovulatory cycle.

Ovulation induction agent with intrauterine inseminations (IUI)

For women who have unexplained infertility, cervical factor, mild male factor or mild endometriosis, clomiphene citrate ovulation induction with IUI treatment is appropriate treatment. This treatment involves the administration of clomiphene citrate at a dose of 100 mg between cycle days 3 and 7. An ovulation predictor kit is used to test the urine beginning on cycle day 11. Once a LH surge is identified, plans are made to perform the IUI. If 3 months of treatment proves unsuccessful then the treatment plan may be reassessed and may include a laparoscopy/hysteroscopy or moving on to more aggressive treatment involving FSH injections with intrauterine inseminations. Like all interventions, the success rate of clomiphene citrate–IUI treatment is influenced by the age of the woman. Women over the age of 35 might benefit from aggressive ovulation induction with FSH as part of IUI treatment.

> *Recommended dosage:* The dose of clomiphene citrate is 100 mg on cycle days 3–7. The patient should be instructed to use an ovulation predictor kit beginning on cycle day 11. When the test turns positive, a single insemination treatment is done the following day. In our experience, approximately 90% of patients will have an LH surge detected between cycle days 11 and 15. An alternative is to perform vaginal ultrasound examinations beginning cycle day 12 and when a dominant follicle is 18 mm or larger the ovulation can be triggered with an injection of human chorionic gonadotropin (hCG) (10 000 IU) and the insemination is scheduled 36 hours later.

Pregnancy rate: 8–10% per cycle.

OTHER MEDICATIONS THAT CAN BE USED WITH CLOMIPHENE CITRATE

In some women with ovulatory dysfunction, other medications may be considered which can be administered by themselves or in addition to clomiphene citrate.

Oral hypoglycemic agents

For decades polycystic ovary syndrome (PCOS) or chronic anovulation has remained a poorly understood disease. Over the past few years, significant advances have been made that have greatly improved our understanding of this disorder. It is now believed that insulin resistance plays a central role in the pathogenesis of PCOS. Insulin resistance is a condition in which the action of insulin is hampered either by a defective insulin receptor or post-receptor defect. With insulin resistance, higher circulating levels of insulin are necessary to maintain normal glucose homeostasis. Hyperinsulinism can explain many of the associated findings of PCOS. Insulin increases ovarian and adrenal androgen production, decreases the production of sex hormone binding globulin and stimulates the pituitary secretion of LH. All of this leads to an androgenic *milieu* that interferes with the normal follicular development and ovulation. Insulin resistance is a metabolic disorder and ovulatory dysfunction is only one of its manifestations. Other abnormalities associated with insulin resistance include Type II diabetes, hypertension, dyslipidemia, centripetal obesity and an increased risk of cardiovascular disease.

Any woman who presents with ovulatory dysfunction and has symptoms of hyperandrogenism should be tested for serum androgens (DHEAS, 17-OH-progesterone, testosterone). In addition, she should have an assessment of the glucose metabolism with fasting insulin and glucose levels. The diagnosis of insulin resistance has been a subject of debate. One group of investigators concluded that a fasting glucose to insulin ratio of less than 4.5 is compatible with a diagnosis of insulin resistance[19]. If the fasting blood sugar is greater than 110 mg/dl glucose intolerance should be suspected and a 2-hour glucose tolerance test should be done to rule out diabetes mellitus. Patients with insulin resistance are at greater risk for the development of gestational diabetes and Type II diabetes. Many individuals with insulin resistance are also overweight. Exercise and good nutrition should be stressed since weight loss will help to improve the insulin resistance and decrease the chances of developing diabetes.

Patients with adult-onset diabetes mellitus have been treated effectively with oral hypoglycemic agents, such as metformin. Metformin improves the actions of insulin in several ways. It increases the uptake of glucose into fat and muscle cells. In addition, it decreases intestinal absorption of glucose and reduces hepatic gluconeogenesis. There are published data that have confirmed that metformin improves the insulin resistance in patients with PCOS, which results in a correction of the ovulatory dysfunction[61–63]. This has been a significant breakthrough in the treatment of PCOS. Many women with PCOS respond poorly to clomiphene citrate and have to be treated with injectable gonadotropins. A previous study reported on 22 women who had chronic oligomenorrhea (six or fewer cycles per year) or amenorrhea. A total of 21 of 22 (95.7%) established normal menstrual function after 6 months of metformin treatment[62]. In another study, metformin was administered to patients who failed to ovulate with clomiphene citrate. After 5 weeks of metformin treatment, 12 of 35 (34%) patients ovulated. Twenty-one of the remaining patients were then treated with clomiphene citrate (in addition to the metformin). A total of 19 of the 21 (90%) patients ovulated on the combined treatment. Therefore, 94% of patients who had previously failed to respond to clomiphene citrate alone ovulated with metformin treatment[61]. It can be concluded that metformin is a useful therapeutic agent to correct the ovulatory dysfunction associated with PCOS.

Evaluation: Perform standard work-up for anovulation. Check fasting glucose and insulin. A glucose to insulin ratio of < 4.5 suggests insulin resistance. However, this is not an absolute prerequisite to metformin treatment. Metformin treatment may be considered in any patient with signs of PCOS. If the fasting blood sugar is greater than 110 mg/dl, perform a 2-hour glucose tolerance test to rule out diabetes. Renal studies (creatinine, BUN) and liver function tests (SGOT, SGPT) should also be obtained. One potential risk of metformin treatment is lactic acidosis. The incidence of this side-effect is increased in those with renal or hepatic dysfunction.

Recommended dosage: Metformin is available in 500-mg tablets. Initiation of metformin should be done in a gradual fashion to decrease the incidence of side-effects. One tablet (500 mg) should be taken daily for 1 week, then one tablet twice a day for 1 week, then one tablet three times a day (1500 mg per day). The medication should be taken with meals. The effective dose of metformin is 500 mg p.o. t.i.d.

Side-effects: Gastrointestinal symptoms, including nausea, vomiting, diarrhea, bloating, and flatulence, occur in 30% of patients who take metformin. These side-effects are usually temporary. Lactic acidosis is a serious metabolic disorder that may be increased in those with renal and/or hepatic dysfunction. Metformin is a schedule B drug but should be discontinued when pregnancy is established. Metformin does not cause hypoglycemia.

Clinical application

Long-term treatment   In some cases, long-term treatment with metformin can be considered for up to 6–12 months. This is especially attractive treatment for the woman who is obese or who wants to avoid a multiple pregnancy. For the patient with obesity, good nutrition and an exercise program should be stressed. Weight loss will increase the effectiveness of metformin. The patient should follow-up with the physician periodically every 6–8 weeks. Monitoring for ovulation or with pregnancy tests should be performed to assess treatment efficacy.

Short-term treatment   For those patients who want to move on quickly to treatment. The patient can be treated with a short course of metformin (4–8 weeks) before moving on to clomiphene citrate.

Clomiphene citrate resistance   Even when insulin resistance is suspected, a trial of clomiphene citrate by itself may be considered. Metformin treatment can be started if no response is noted to clomiphene citrate.

Dopaminergic agents

Hyperprolactinemia is a cause of ovulatory dysfunction. A prolactin determination should be obtained on any woman who presents with irregular or absent menstrual periods and/or galactorrhea. It is important that the prolactin level is assessed on a blood sample drawn in the morning (around 10 o'clock) during the follicular phase of the menstrual cycle. At other times of the day, and in the luteal phase, physiological elevations of prolactin can occur. If an elevated prolactin level is found, the assessment should be repeated for verification. If a woman is found to have persistent hyperprolactinemia then a cause should be determined. Hyperprolactinemia can be secondary to previous breast surgery, neck trauma, medication use, renal insufficiency, a pituitary tumor and hypothyroidism. Any woman with unexplained hyperprolactinemia when associated with ovulatory dysfunction should have a MRI of the head to rule out a pituitary tumor. Several dopaminergic agents are available to correct the hyperprolactinemia (e.g. bromocriptine, cabergoline). Many times, these agents are effective by themselves in correcting the ovulatory dysfunction. In a previous review reporting on 22 clinical trials, it was noted that 80% of women with hyperprolactinemia had restoration of their menstrual function[64]. On average, menstrual function returned 5.7 weeks after treatment was started. If the woman fails to develop normal ovulatory cycles despite the establishment of a normal prolactin level then the clinician may consider adding clomiphene citrate or another ovulation induction agent to the treatment regimen.

Some patients have hyperprolactinemia despite normal menstrual cycles. There are different species of prolactin that circulate in the blood stream, some active others not. Most likely in these situations the majority of the circulating prolactin is the inactive variety, has no biological significance and does not necessitate treatment.

Available agents and doses

- *Bromocriptine (Parlodel®)* Available in 2.5-mg tablets. Start with half a tablet (1.25 mg) q.h.s. for 1 week then increase up to one tablet (2.5 mg) q.h.s. Repeat prolactin level in 2–3 weeks. If the prolactin level is increased the dose can be increased in an incremental fashion.

- *Cabergoline (Dostinex®)* Available in 0.5-mg tablets. Start with one tablet (0.5 mg) twice a week. Dose may be increased by 0.25 mg twice weekly to less than or equal to 1 mg twice a week, depending on the serum prolactin level. Do not increase dose more often than every 4 weeks.

Side-effects: The more common side-effects include gastrointestinal upset, fatigue, dizziness, and nasal stuffiness.

Dexamethasone

Dexamethasone can be considered for the anovulatory woman (who does not have evidence of insulin resistance) who fails to respond to increasing doses of clomiphene citrate or is noted to have an elevated DHEAS level. An elevated DHEAS level may suggest an attenuated adrenal enzyme deficiency. Other causes include an adrenal tumor and Cushing's syndrome, which must be considered but are, nonetheless, rare. The administration of dexamethasone will decrease the adrenal androgen contribution to the pool of androgens. In some cases, this will be enough to improve the response to clomiphene citrate. Dexamethasone should be administered at night at a dose of 0.5 mg. One month after starting the dexamethasone, a morning cortisol level should be checked. If the cortisol level is less than 3 μg/dl this suggests significant depression of cortisol synthesis by the adrenal gland, which could interfere with a stress response by the adrenal gland. In this circumstance, the dose or frequency of administration should be decreased. The use of dexamethasone should be avoided during pregnancy.

Recommended reading

- Yen SSC, Jaffe RB, Barbieri RL. *Reproductive Endocrinology*. Philadelphia: W.B. Saunders Company, 1999
- Speroff L, Glass RH, Kase NG. *Clinical Gynecologic Endocrinology and Infertility*. Baltimore: Williams & Wilkins, 1999
- American College of Obstetricians and Gynecologists (ACOG). *Managing the Anovulatory State: Medical Induction of Ovulation*. Technical Bulletin Number 197, September 1994

8.

Progesterone therapy

Progesterone is an ovarian hormone that plays an important role in reproduction. This fact is not refuted; however, controversy exists as to whether a deficiency of progesterone can be a cause of infertility or a pregnancy loss. Another area of controversy concerns the role of progesterone supplementation, including the indications and the optimal method of administration. This chapter will provide a better understanding of this topic.

THE NORMAL MENSTRUAL CYCLE

The objective of the menstrual cycle is the ovulation of an oocyte that can be fertilized and the development of an endometrium that is conducive to implantation. This is dependent on the complex interaction between the hypothalamus, pituitary gland, the ovary and the endometrium. Ultimately, it is the estradiol and progesterone produced by the ovary that impact on the endometrium. The first stage of the menstrual cycle, termed the *proliferative phase* is an estrogen-dominant phase. Estradiol is the most potent estrogen that is produced which results from the aromatization of androgens by the granulosa cells of the developing follicles. Estradiol stimulates the growth of the endometrium. Following ovulation, the granulosa cells in the collapsed follicle sequester cholesterol, which is the precursor to progesterone. Progesterone dominates this stage of the menstrual cycle, which is termed the *secretory phase*. Progesterone acts as an anti-estrogen and arrests the estrogen-induced growth of the endometrium and causes maturation of the endometrium, which will allow implantation to occur. In addition, ovarian production of progesterone is important in supporting the pregnancy up until the 7–9th week, at which time placental production takes over.

PROGESTERONE SECRETION DURING PREGNANCY

During a normal pregnancy, progesterone levels plateau during the first trimester (10–30 ng/ml), then begin rising gradually in the early second trimester and reach maximal levels at term (100–150 ng/ml). It had been proposed that a progesterone level during the early part of pregnancy might be predictive of the viability of the pregnancy. However, studies have confirmed that a progesterone level by itself is not accurate in predicting the outcome of a pregnancy unless it is significantly depressed[65,66]. In a previous study, the authors confirmed that if the serum progesterone level was below 5 ng/ml there was < 1% chance the pregnancy was viable[67]. The hallmark for assessing the viability of the pregnancy relies on the knowledge of the gestational age, rate of rise and level of the β-hCG titers, and vaginal ultrasonography findings. In addition to this assessment, some clinicians like to use a serum progesterone level, as well. However, during the early stages of pregnancy, if a low progesterone level is encountered it does not mean that there is a progesterone deficiency that needs to be treated. Rather, a low progesterone level along with poorly rising β-hCG titers may be indicative of a non-viable pregnancy.

> **Routine progesterone monitoring during pregnancy is *not* necessary. Further, there is no indication for progesterone supplementation when a low progesterone level is identified.**

LUTEAL PHASE DEFICIENCY: DOES IT EXIST?

In years past, there was emphasis on luteal phase deficiency as a cause of infertility and recurrent miscarriages. It was theorized that some women may be ovulating and having regular menstrual cycles but that the progesterone secreted during the luteal phase is insufficient to mature the endometrium for implantation or unable to support a pregnancy. There were two approaches to the evaluation of the adequacy of the luteal phase. The first was measuring a mid-luteal phase progesterone level. If the progesterone level was below 10 ng/ml then this was suggestive of a progesterone deficiency. The major difficulty with using progesterone levels in this fashion is that progesterone is secreted in pulses every 2–3 hours, which will interfere with the interpretation of a single level[68]. The more popular technique to assess the adequacy of the luteal phase was an endometrial biopsy performed late in the luteal phase. It was thought that the endometrial biopsy represented a bioassay of all of the progesterone that was secreted during the luteal phase. Progesterone causes day-to-day changes in the endometrium that can be appreciated histologically. A luteal phase deficiency was established if there was at least a 3-day lag between the histological date of the endometrial biopsy and the chronological date of the menstrual cycle (established retrospectively with the knowledge of the onset of the next menses and assuming a 14-day luteal phase). From a theoretical standpoint, this makes good sense, but there are problems using with the endometrial biopsy for this purpose, including:

(1) Uncertainty when the menstrual period begins which may interfere with the establishment of the chronological day;

(2) Interobserver variation in the pathological interpretation of the biopsy;

(3) The false premise that the luteal phase is 14 days in length, which can actually range between 13 and 16 days;

(4) 20% of fertile women will have an out-of-phase endometrial biopsy.

The data published to date raise questions about the diagnosis of luteal phase deficiency[15–17]. Taking this into consideration, plus the unreliability of the testing and the lack of proof of treatment efficacy, we do not feel that assessment of the luteal phase should be a part of the infertility evaluation.

The current understanding is that luteal phase deficiency is *not* a clinical entity. Furthermore, assessment of the luteal phase is not considered a part of the routine infertility evaluation.

INDICATIONS FOR PROGESTERONE SUPPLEMENTATION

There are situations when the clinician may consider progesterone supplementation, which is discussed below.

Recurrent miscarriages

The clinician may consider supplemental progesterone for the patient with recurrent miscarriages. It is important that all couples who have experienced two or more miscarriages undergo a recurrent miscarriage work-up (Table 8.1).

Table 8.1   Recurrent miscarriage work-up

1. Rule out environmental exposures and lifestyle issues
2. Assessment of ovarian function
   - Menstrual history
   - Cycle 3 – FSH, estradiol, TSH
3. Examination of uterine cavity by one of the following:
   - Hysterosalpingogram
   - Sonohysterogram
   - Hysteroscopy
4. Autoimmune work-up
   - Anticardiolipin antibodies
   - Lupus anticoagulant
5. Chromosomal
   - Karyotypes on both partners

If the work-up is negative, the couple can be offered empiric progesterone supplementation. It must be emphasized to the couple that there are no documented studies demonstrating the efficacy of this treatment in preventing future pregnancy losses. However, progesterone is a safe treatment with minimal risks to the mother and the fetus. The progesterone should be started 3–4 days after a temperature shift with a basal body temperature chart or following a urinary LH surge determined by an ovulation predictor kit. The progesterone can be continued until the 10th week of pregnancy. Patients should be counseled that progesterone administration could delay the onset of a menstrual period even if pregnancy is not established.

IVF treatment

It is standard that all women undergoing IVF treatment receive progesterone supplementation during the luteal phase. However, an investigation has not been carried out to analyze whether progesterone is even necessary for IVF patients. It has been hypothesized that deficient progesterone production may result from the down-regulation with a GnRH agonist, the disruption of the follicular granulosa cells during the egg retrieval and/or the high estrogen levels that are encountered during this treatment. There is some controversy as to which is the best route of administration, oral, vaginal or intramuscular injection. We generally will continue the supplementation until fetal viability is confirmed by vaginal ultrasound that is generally performed between the 6th and 7th week of gestation. However, a previous study concluded that progesterone can be safely discontinued on the day of the first positive pregnancy test[69].

Women undergoing egg donation or gestational carrier treatment are also treated with progesterone supplements. Since these women are either in ovarian failure or on a GnRH agonist there is no ovarian hormone production. Therefore, estrogen and progesterone are administered together and are continued until the 10th week of pregnancy.

Removal of a corpus luteum

Following ovulation and during the early part of pregnancy, hemorrhage can occur into the corpus luteum that can result in intraperitoneal bleeding and severe abdominal pain. In some situations, surgical intervention may be indicated. Surgical treatment could simply involve cauterization of the bleeding site, removal of the corpus luteum or an oophorectomy. The corpus luteum is responsible for progesterone production until the 7–9th weeks of pregnancy.

Therefore, if there is any disruption or removal of the corpus luteum during the early part of pregnancy, progesterone supplementation would be indicated and should be continued until the 10th week of pregnancy.

PROGESTERONE AGENTS

Progesterone can be administered orally, vaginally and by intramuscular injection. It is our opinion that the vaginal route is the optimal way to administer progesterone. While it is true that higher serum levels are achieved by intramuscular injection, the endometrial tissue levels are seven-fold higher with vaginal administration as compared to intramuscular injection[70]. Following its absorption via the vaginal route of administration, progesterone is circulated directly to the uterus before it is distributed and diluted in the systemic circulation. This is referred to as the 'first-pass effect' which maximizes delivery of the hormone to the target organ. There are several vaginal progesterone preparations available including Crinone® and progesterone vaginal suppositories that need to be made up by the pharmacist. Prometrium® capsules are also available for oral administration but we have been using it successively with vaginal administration as well.

Available progesterone agents

Vaginal preparations:
➤ Crinone® – 90 mg (one application) q.d.
➤ Vaginal suppositories[†] – 100 mg b.i.d
➤ Prometrium® (micronized progesterone) – 200 mg b.i.d.

Note: For vaginal preparations (except Crinone®) patients should be instructed to remain supine for 20 minutes after inserting the preparation into the vagina.

Oral preparations:
➤ Prometrium® (micronized progesterone) – 100 mg t.i.d. – should be taken with meals to enhance absorption

Intramuscular injections:
➤ Progesterone-in-oil – available in 10-cc bottles (50 mg/cc); administer 50 mg q.d. (1 cc) by intramuscular injection on a daily basis

[†] These preparations are not as readily available since they have to be made up special by the pharmacist in advance.

9.

Methotrexate therapy

In the past, the treatment for an ectopic pregnancy was almost exclusively a surgical approach. Over 10 years ago, methotrexate was introduced as a medical treatment for this condition. Initially, methotrexate was administered to women who had persistent trophoblastic tissue that remained in the Fallopian tube following a salpingostomy. Over the past decade, there have several published studies demonstrating the effectiveness and safety of methotrexate when used as primary treatment for an ectopic pregnancy[71]. In today's medical practice, medical treatment for an ectopic pregnancy offers an alternative to surgery.

EPIDEMIOLOGY

Approximately 1% of all pregnancies do not implant in the uterine cavity and are ectopic in location. The majority (95%) of ectopic pregnancies are located in the Fallopian tube and the remainder are located in the ovary, cervical canal and the abdominal cavity. Risk factors for an ectopic pregnancy include: a previous pelvic infection, current or previous use of an intrauterine device (IUD), tubal reconstructive surgery, infertility, increased maternal age, *in utero* exposure to DES and a previous ectopic pregnancy. Women who have had a previous ectopic pregnancy have a 10% chance of a recurrent ectopic pregnancy with a future pregnancy.

CLINICAL PRESENTATION OF AN ECTOPIC PREGNANCY

The classic symptoms of an ectopic pregnancy are amenorrhea, unilateral abdominal pain and abnormal vaginal bleeding. However, these symptoms only result when the ectopic pregnancy is at an advanced stage. Monitoring with vaginal ultrasonography and serial β-hCG titers during the early part of pregnancy have helped us to diagnose an ectopic pregnancy at an early stage before symptoms develop. An ectopic pregnancy can be diagnosed when the vaginal ultrasound demonstrates the presence of a gestational sac outside the uterine cavity. A presumed ectopic can be considered when there is lack of visualization of a gestational sac in the uterine cavity by vaginal ultrasound at 6 weeks of gestation or when the β-hCG titer is > 2000 mIU/ml. An ectopic pregnancy should also be suspected when the β-hCG titers are not rising normally. As a general rule, the mean doubling time for the β-hCG titer is 48 hours. Studies analyzing the rate of rise of the titers have confirmed that 85% of viable pregnancies rise at least 66% over 48 hours. Conversely, 15% of viable pregnancies rise less than 66% in the 48-hour period[72,73].

MANAGEMENT OPTIONS

The clinician now has several treatment options to choose from for the management of an ectopic pregnancy. The appropriate treatment will depend on the presentation and other considerations.

Observation

Patients who are suspected of having an ectopic pregnancy and are clinically stable should have the β-hCG titer repeated in 2–3 days. If the titer decreases, then the ectopic pregnancy could be undergoing spontaneous resolution and observation is the indicated treatment, as long as the titers continue to decrease and the patient remains clinically stable. Spontaneous resolution is more likely to occur when the β-hCG titers are lower[74]. A previous study confirmed that 90% of abnormal pregnancies with β-hCG titers less than 200 mIU/ml resolved without intervention[75]. It is important to realize that even if the titers are decreasing, tubal rupture can still occur. For this reason, any complaints of abdominal pain experienced by the patient should be investigated.

Surgical treatment

If the patient is unstable or there is concern of tubal rupture, then surgical treatment is indicated. For other presentations, a medical or surgical approach can be considered. There are advantages to surgical treatment for an ectopic pregnancy. A laparoscopic examination allows a definitive diagnosis to be established and it provides the surgeon the opportunity to determine the condition of the tubes and ovaries. This information is helpful for the woman who has a history of infertility. If a woman has experienced a second ectopic pregnancy in the same tube she should be counseled on the option of a salpingectomy. If the ectopic pregnancy is unruptured, then conservative surgery with a linear salpingostomy is indicated. When compared to medical treatment, conservative surgery results in a more rapid decrease in β-hCG titers and earlier resolution. The major disadvantages of surgery are the risks associated with the anesthesia and the surgery itself, and the time needed for postoperative recovery.

Medical treatment with methotrexate

Treatment with methotrexate offers another treatment option for patients. When it was originally introduced it was used to treat women who had rising or plateauing β-hCG titers following conservative surgical treatment. Since then there have been several reports describing the safety and efficacy of methotrexate treatment as initial treatment for an ectopic pregnancy[76–79].

Action

Methotrexate is a folic acid antagonist that binds to the catalytic site of dihydrofolate reductase, which interrupts the synthesis of the purine nucleotide thymidilate and amino acids, serine and methionine. Thus, methotrexate interferes with deoxyribonucleic acid (DNA) synthesis and cell multiplication. Actively proliferating trophoblastic tissue is sensitive to this effect of methotrexate, which forms the rationale for its use in the treatment of ectopic pregnancy as well as gestational trophoblastic disease.

Indications for methotrexate administration

A woman who may be considered a candidate for methotrexate administration is one who:

(1) Has a documented gestational sac outside of the uterine cavity;

(2) Has an ectopic pregnancy in a location (i.e. the cervix, cornua, and ovary) that is not amenable to surgical treatment;

(3) Is a poor operative risk;

(4) Has a suspected ectopic pregnancy:

   (a) abnormally rising β-hCG titers;

   (b) no evidence of an intrauterine pregnancy by vaginal ultrasound when the β-hCG titer has reached 2000 mIU/ml and/or at 6 weeks of gestation;

(c) no villae identified in the tissue removed with a dilatation and curettage and rising or plateauing β-hCG titers during the postoperative period;

(5) Has rising or plateauing β-hCG titers following a linear salpingostomy.

Contraindications for methotrexate administration

A woman who is not considered a candidate for methotrexate administration is one who:

(1) Is clinically unstable (decreased hematocrit, evidence of hemorrhage or worsening abdominal pain);

(2) Has impaired renal and liver function, thrombocytopenia or leukopenia;

(3) Has a co-existing viable intrauterine pregnancy;

(4) Is non-compliant;

(5) Is breastfeeding;

(6) Has any of the following:

  (a) history of alcohol abuse;

  (b) active pulmonary disease;

  (c) peptic ulcer disease;

  (d) liver disease;

(7) Has gestational sac ($\geq$ 3.5 cm), β-hCG titer > 10 000 mIU/ml or fetal heart activity (relative contraindications).

Pretreatment evaluation

The following are prerequisites that must be met before treatment with methotrexate can be considered:

(1) A medical consultation with a history and physical examination;

(2) A vaginal ultrasound examination;

(3) Baseline laboratory work, including:

  (a) blood type and screen with the administration of Rhogam®, if indicated;

  (b) CBC;

  (d) platelet count;

  (e) SGOT;

(f) β-hCG titer;

(g) creatinine;

(4) Determination the patient's height and weight;

(5) A signed consent form prior to the initiation of treatment.

Administration

Methotrexate is a chemotherapeutic drug and special care must be taken with the administration and handling of this medication. We recommend that you talk about these issues with a pharmacist before using this medication. The

---

Calculating the dose of methotrexate

The recommended dosage of methotrexate is 50 mg/m^2

Step 1   Calculate the surface area (m^2)

$$m^2 = \sqrt{\frac{\text{Height (inches)} \times \text{Weight (lbs)}}{3131}}$$

(Mosteller RD. Simplified calculation of body surface area. *N Engl J Med* 1987;317:1098)

Step 2   Calculate the total dose (mg) of methotrexate to be administered

Dose (mg) = surface area (m^2) × 50 mg/m^2

Step 3   Give these calculations to the pharmacist to verify the accuracy. The pharmacist will dispense the medication and the volume of the injection should not exceed more than 2 cc per injection site.

Sample calculations for a patient who weighs 152 lbs and is 5′ 2″ (62″) tall

Step 1   Calculate the surface area (m^2)

$$m^2 = \sqrt{\frac{62 \text{ inches} \times 152 \text{ lbs}}{3131}} = 1.73 \text{ m}^2$$

Step 2   Calculate the total dose (mg)

Dose (mg) = 1.73 m^2 × 50 mg/m^2 = 86.5 mg

Step 3   Methotrexate is available in a concentration of 25 mg/cc. For this particular patient, a total of 3.5 cc would be necessary to administer the 86.5 mg. This volume would be divided into two equal injections of 1.75 cc (44 mg each).

---

standard dose of methotrexate to be administered is 50 mg/m^2. The dose is based on surface area (m^2), which is calculated from the patient's height and weight (see sample calculation). We recommend that the pharmacist verify the surface-area calculation and the dose to be administered. The injection is administered by intramuscular injection and is well tolerated by the patients.

Patient instructions

Following the injection and until there is resolution the patient should be instructed to avoid:

- Alcohol
- Folic acid and vitamins that contain folic acid
- Exposure to the sun, sun lamp and tanning salons
- Non-steroidal inflammatory agents
- Immunizations
- Intercourse

See page 122 for Patient Instruction Sheet.

Post-injection follow-up

Following the administration of methotrexate a repeat β-hCG titer will be measured 4 and 7 days after the injection. In most cases, the titer obtained 4 days after the injection will continue to rise when compared to the titer obtained on the day of injection. The delayed effectiveness following the injection is because it takes several days before the methotrexate gets incorporated into the cell cycle of the trophoblastic tissue.

- If there is *greater* than a 15% decline between titers post-injection days 4 and 7, then weekly β-hCG titers are obtained and followed until they are negative. During follow-up if there is less than a 15% reduction between weekly titers then a repeat dose of methotrexate can be given

- If there is *less* than a 15% decline between titers post-injection days 4 and 7, a second dose of methotrexate 50 mg/m^2 can be administered and the titers are again assessed on days 4 and 7 after the injection

- If there is *less* than a 15% decline between titers on post-treatment days 4 and 7, a third dose of methotrexate 50 mg/m^2 can be administered

- Alternatively, laparoscopic evaluation may be an alternative

Because of the risk of tubal rupture, intercourse should be avoided until the β-hCG titer has become negative. However, for those patients who choose to have intercourse they should be counseled to use contraception.

Side-effects

Side-effects usually do not appear until 2–7 days after administration. Side-effects include nausea, vomiting, stomatitis, diarrhea, dizziness and loss of appetite. Rarely, methotrexate can cause leukopenia and/or thrombocytopenia. Other very uncommon side-effects include hair loss, skin rash, dizziness and liver dysfunction. Abdominal pain is another symptom that can be noted after administration of the drug[78,79]. This symptom is most likely the result of separation of the ectopic pregnancy from the tube. Others have theorized that some abdominal symptoms may be secondary to a transient toxic effect of methotrexate on the gastrointestinal tract. However, depending on the severity of the pain, the patient should be evaluated to rule out tubal rupture with a pelvic examination, vaginal ultrasound and a β-hCG titer.

Clinical results

There have been several reports investigating the use of methotrexate for the treatment of ectopic pregnancy. The largest study reported on 320 women who underwent methotrexate treatment for an ectopic pregnancy[80]. Following medical treatment, 91% of patients had resolution of the ectopic pregnancies. A total of 81% responded to one injection, 17% required two injections and 2% required three injections. The mean time until resolution was 5 weeks. The medical treatment was well tolerated with few side-effects. The following factors were not predictors of success: the woman's age or parity, the size of the ectopic pregnancy, and the presence or absence of fluid in the peritoneal cavity. Fetal heart activity was present in 12% of the successfully treated cases and 30% of those in which methotrexate treatment was unsuccessful. Regression analysis confirmed that only the initial β-hCG titer was predictive of success, which is presented in Table 9.1. From this study it can be concluded that the pretreatment β-hCG titer and the presence of fetal heart activity are factors that influence the success of methotrexate treatment.

Table 9.1 The success of methotrexate treatment related to initial β-hCG titer. Modified from Lipscomb, et al.[80]

Initial β-hCG titer	Success	Failure	Success rate (95% CI)	
< 1000	118	2	98%	(96–100)
1000–1999	40	3	93%	(85–100)
2000–4999	90	8	92%	(86–97)
5000–9999	39	6	87%	(79–98)
10 000–14 999	18	4	82%	(65–98)
≥15 000	15	7	68%	(49–88)

CONCLUSION

Medical treatment with methotrexate offers another treatment option for patients with ectopic pregnancies. In selected cases, it has demonstrated its efficacy and safety, and it is cost-effective when compared to a surgical approach.

> **Recommended reading**
> - American College of Obstetricians and Gynecologists (ACOG). *Clinical Management Guidelines for Obstetrician-Gynecologists; Medical Management of Tubal Pregnancy*. Practice Bulletin Number 3, December 1998

METHOTREXATE ADMINISTRATION FLOW SHEET

Name_____ Physician_____ Height_____

Date of birth_____ LMP_____ Weight_____

Diagnosis: ❏ Proven ectopic ❏ Presumed ectopic ❏ Persistent ectopic

Day 0: CBC: nl abnl **SGOT:** nl abnl **CREATININE:** nl abnl **Blood type_____**

REPEAT: CBC: nl abnl **SGOT:** nl abnl **CREATININE:** nl abnl

---

Calculating the dose of methotrexate

$$\text{Dose (mg)} = \text{surface area (m}^2) \times 50 \text{ mg/m}^2$$

$$= \sqrt{\frac{\text{(inches)} \times \quad \text{(lbs)}}{3131}} \times 50 = \text{_____} \text{ mg}$$

Date	β-hCG titer	Ultrasound results	MTX Dose	Comments

Protocol for following β-hCG titers after methotrexate administration:

Following the administration of methotrexate a repeat β-hCG titer will be measured 4 and 7 days after the injection. In most cases, the titer obtained 4 days after the injection will continue to rise.

- If there is *greater* than a 15% decline between titers post-injection days 4 and 7, then weekly β-hCG titers are obtained and followed until they are negative. During follow-up, if there is less than a 15% reduction between weekly titers then a repeat dose of methotrexate can be given.
- If there is *less* than a 15% decline between post-injection days 4 and 7 titers, a second dose of methotrexate 50 mg/m^2 can be administered and the titers are again assessed on days 4 and 7 after the injection. Repeat screening blood work.
- If there is *less* than a 15% decline between titers post-treatment days 4 and 7, a third dose of methotrexate 50 mg/m^2 can be administered. Alternatively, laparoscopic evaluation may be an alternative.

PATIENT INSTRUCTIONS FOLLOWING METHOTREXATE ADMINISTRATION

For 2 weeks following the injection, you should:

- Not drink alcohol

- Not take folic acid or vitamins that contain folic acid

- Avoid excessive exposure to the sun, sun lamp and tanning

- Avoid the use of aspirin and aspirin-like compounds, including: Advil®, Motrin®, Ibuprofen®, Naprosyn®, Aleve®, etc.

- Avoid any immunizations or vaccines since methotrexate can affect the immune system

- Avoid intercourse until resolution

Continue with your normal activities and if you have any symptoms, including abdominal pain, pain at the injection site or other symptoms, please contact us immediately.

10.
Consent forms

Informed consent is at the foundation of medical practice and should precede any medical or surgical intervention. Informed consent is not just having the patient sign a consent form, but rather it is a process that involves extensive discussions with the patient about the risks, benefits and alternatives to the proposed treatment or procedure. The signing of the consent is symbolic and represents a completion of the process. To this end, it is important for the physician to document in the chart any discussions that took place and pamphlets or other materials that were given to the patient in relation to the proposed intervention. For additional information regarding the informed consent process, the reader is referred to two excellent publications by the American College of Obstetricians and Gynecologists (ACOG): *ACOG Committee Opinion: Ethical Dimensions of Informed Consent*, Number 108, May 1992 and *The Assistant: Informed Consent*, Department of Professional Liability, Number 4, 1998.

We have provided several sample consents forms for review for the following procedures and treatments:

Laparoscopy
Hysteroscopy
Hysterosalpingogram
Sonohysterogram
Endometrial biopsy
Clomiphene citrate
Methotrexate

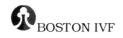BOSTON IVF

CONSENT FORM
FOR A LAPAROSCOPY

A laparoscopy is an outpatient surgical procedure that is performed to diagnose and treat conditions of the pelvic organs such as infertility, pelvic pain, pelvic masses and other disorders.

PROCEDURE

When you arrive at the surgical suite, an anesthesiologist will place an intravenous line. You will then be taken to the operating room and general anesthesia will be administered. Then a pelvic examination is performed and an instrument is inserted into the uterine cavity that allows manipulation of the uterus during the procedure. Next, a small incision (1–2 cm) is made just below the navel through which a small telescopic instrument, called a laparoscope, is inserted into the abdominal cavity. Usually, one to three additional incisions are made in the lower abdomen through which other instruments can be inserted. After all the instruments are in place, a systematic inspection of the pelvis is performed including an examination of the uterus, Fallopian tubes, ovaries and all other surrounding organs. If either pelvic adhesions or endometriosis is identified, a decision may be made to treat these conditions at the time of the surgery with the laser, electrocautery or scissors. If a cyst or a mass is identified in the region of the ovary or the Fallopian tube, a decision may be made to remove it. At the end of the procedure, a non-toxic colored dye may be injected into the uterine cavity to determine if the Fallopian tubes are open. Depending on the findings, the procedure may take 1–3 hours to complete.

POSTOPERATIVE CARE

After the procedure has been completed, you will spend a few hours in the recovery room and then be discharged home. Since you may be drowsy following the procedure, it is important that someone is available to transport you home and be with you. It is not uncommon to have some vaginal spotting and mild lower abdominal cramping following the procedure. You will be prescribed a medication to provide pain relief following the procedure. You should plan on resting the following day after the surgery. There are no restrictions on showering or bathing. You should refrain from intercourse for 5 days following the procedure. If at any time during the postoperative course, you develop any fever, chills, severe abdominal pain, heavy vaginal bleeding, or any other symptoms, you should call your physician immediately.

COMPLICATIONS

The reported complication rate following a laparoscopy is less than 1–2%. Because sharp instruments are used to insert the instruments, there is the potential to injure vital organs, some of which include the intestines, bladder, ureters, uterus, major blood vessels and other pelvic organs. Injury could necessitate hospitalization and the performance of additional surgery. Additional surgery could include a life-saving hysterectomy and/or resection of damaged intestine with a colostomy. Death is a very rare complication following this procedure.

ACKNOWLEDGEMENT OF INFORMED CONSENT

I acknowledge that I have read and understand this written material. I understand the purpose, risks, benefits and alternatives of the surgery. I am aware that there may be other risks and complications not discussed that may occur. I also understand that during the course of the procedure, unforeseen conditions may be revealed requiring the performance of additional procedures. I also understand that technical problems with the instrumentation may prevent the completion of the surgery. I acknowledge that no guarantees or promises have been made to me concerning the results of this procedure or any treatment that may be required as a result of this procedure. I have been given the opportunity to ask questions which have been answered to my satisfaction.

I consent to the performance of the procedure described above.

_____   _____

Signature of Patient   Signature of Physician

_____

Printed Name

_____

Date of Birth

_____

Date

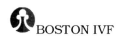BOSTON IVF

CONSENT FORM
FOR A HYSTEROSCOPY

A hysteroscopy is an outpatient surgical procedure that allows visualization of the uterine cavity. This procedure allows the diagnosis of uterine abnormalities that could be a cause of infertility or abnormal bleeding.

PROCEDURE

When you arrive at the surgical suite, an anesthesiologist will start an intravenous line. You will then be taken to the operating room and the anesthesia will be administered. You will be placed in the same position as you are for a pelvic exam. After the cervical canal is dilated, a small telescope-like instrument, called a hysteroscope, is inserted into the uterine cavity. Distension of the cavity with a solution then allows examination of the uterine cavity. If any abnormalities are identified, such as a polyp, fibroid, uterine septum, or intrauterine adhesions, other instruments (including the laser, cautery or microscissors) can be used through the operating channel of the hysteroscope and an attempt can be made to treat the condition. In some cases, following the hysteroscopy, a uterine curettage is performed which involves the placement of a small instrument, called a curette, into the uterine cavity, which allows sampling of endometrial tissue.

POSTOPERATIVE CARE

After the procedure has been completed, you will spend a few hours in the recovery room and then be discharged home. Since you may be drowsy follow-ing the procedure, it is important that someone is available to transport you home and be with you. It is not uncommon to have some vaginal bleeding and mild lower abdominal cramping following the procedure. You should plan on resting the following day after the surgery. There are no restrictions on shower-ing or bathing. You should refrain from intercourse and douching for 5 days following the procedure. If during the postoperative course you develop any fever, chills, severe abdominal pain, heavy vaginal bleeding, or any other abnormal symptoms, call your physician immediately.

COMPLICATIONS

The major complication from this procedure is perforation of the wall of the uterus. If this occurs, the procedure is stopped and the injury site may be further examined by a laparoscopy. In most instances, the bleeding at the perforation site is minimal, and the perforation heals without problems. Perforation can result in injury to adjacent organs including the intestines, bladder, ureters, uterus and blood vessels. Injury to these organs could result in a hospitalization and additional surgery to repair the injury. In rare cases, a hysterectomy and removal of tube(s) and ovaries may need to be performed. Death is a very rare complication following a hysteroscopy.

ACKNOWLEDGEMENT OF INFORMED CONSENT

I acknowledge that I have read and understand this written material. I understand the purpose, risks, benefits and alternatives of the surgery. I am aware that there may be other risks and complications not discussed that may occur. I also understand that during the course of the procedure, unforeseen conditions may be revealed requiring the performance of additional procedures. I also understand that technical problems with the instrumentation may prevent the completion of the surgery. I acknowledge that no guarantees or promises have been made to me concerning the results of this procedure or any treatment that may be required as a result of this procedure. I have been given the opportunity to ask questions which have been answered to my satisfaction.

I consent to the performance of the procedure described above by my physician.

_____   _____
Signature of Patient   Signature of Physician

_____
Printed Name

_____
Date of Birth

_____
Date

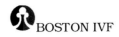 BOSTON IVF

CONSENT FORM FOR A
HYSTEROSALPINGOGRAM

A hysterosalpingogram is an X-ray procedure that is performed to examine the uterine cavity and to determine whether the Fallopian tubes are open. This procedure is commonly performed to identify potential causes of infertility. In addition, it can be performed to examine the uterine cavity in women who have irregular or heavy menstrual periods.

PROCEDURE

This test is performed with the assistance of a radiologist. First, a pelvic examination is performed with insertion of the speculum into the vagina to visualize the cervix. An instrument is attached to the cervix and then a small tube is placed into the cervical canal. Through this tube an iodine-containing solution is injected into the uterine cavity. The progress of the injected solution into the uterine cavity and the Fallopian tubes is followed by viewing a television monitor. Generally, the test is completed within 4–5 minutes. The test can be associated with lower abdominal cramping that subsides after the test is completed.

COMPLICATIONS

The complication rate from this procedure is less than 2%. Some of the complications include the following:

1. ***Pelvic infection*** The performance of this test can result in an infection that could produce lower abdominal pain and fever that develop within a few days following completion of the procedure. A consequence of this infection may be scarred Fallopian tubes and infertility. Infections are more likely to occur in women who have already had a previous pelvic infection and/or damaged tubes. If an infection develops, hospitalization with IV antibiotics and, potentially, surgery may be indicated.

2. ***Allergic reaction*** The contrast medium that is used contains iodine. If you have had any allergic reaction to iodine, a reaction following a radiological procedure [i.e. Cat (CT) scan, intravenous pylogram (IVP)] or if you have had a reaction to fish or shellfish, please notify the physician. This could be suggestive of an iodine allergy.

3. ***Exposure of potential pregnancy*** Despite your perception of a normal menstrual period, there is always the possibility of a potential pregnancy. If

your last menstrual period was abnormal, either delayed or lighter, you should notify your physician.

INSTRUCTIONS FOLLOWING THE TEST

Following the completion of the test you can return to your normal routine. You should avoid intercourse and douching for the next 2 days. If you develop any fever, chills, severe abdominal pain or heavy vaginal bleeding, you should contact the physician immediately.

ACKNOWLEDGEMENT OF INFORMED CONSENT AND AUTHORIZATION

I acknowledge that I have read and understand this written material. I understand the purpose, risks, benefits and alternatives of this procedure. I am aware that there may be other risks and complications not discussed that may occur. I also understand that during the course of the procedure, unforeseen conditions may be revealed requiring the performance of additional procedures. I also understand that technical problems with the instrumentation may prevent the completion of the procedure. I acknowledge that no guarantees or promises have been made to me concerning the results of this procedure or any treatment that may be required as a result of this procedure. I have been given the opportunity to ask questions which have been answered to my satisfaction. I consent to the performance of the procedure described above by my physician.

_____   _____
Signature of Patient   Signature of Physician

_____
Printed Name

_____
Date of Birth

_____
Date

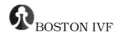BOSTON IVF

CONSENT FORM FOR A
SONOHYSTEROGRAM

A sonohysterogram is a procedure that is performed to examine the uterine cavity. This procedure may help to determine the cause of a woman's infertility or abnormal bleeding. For women with uterine fibroids, the sonohysterogram is helpful to determine whether the fibroids have entered the uterine cavity.

PROCEDURE

The test is performed by a physician. First, a pelvic examination is performed with insertion of the speculum into the vagina to visualize the cervix. Next, a small catheter is inserted through the cervical canal into the uterine cavity. After the catheter is put in place, a vaginal ultrasound probe is inserted into the vagina. Once the uterus is visualized, saline is injected through the catheter into the uterine cavity. The progress of the saline into the uterine cavity is followed by viewing the ultrasound screen. Generally, the test is completed within 4–5 minutes. The test can be associated with mild lower abdominal cramping that subsides after the test is completed.

COMPLICATIONS

The complication rate from this procedure is less than 2%. Some of the risks include the following:

1. **Pelvic infection** The performance of this test can result in an infection that could produce lower abdominal pain and fever that develop within a few days following completion of the procedure. A consequence of this infection may be scarred Fallopian tubes and infertility. Infections are more likely to occur in women who have already had a previous pelvic infection and damaged tubes. If an infection develops, hospitalization with IV antibiotics and, potentially, surgery may be indicated.

2. **Exposure of potential pregnancy** Despite your perception of a normal menstrual period, there is always the possibility of a potential pregnancy. If your last menstrual period was abnormal, either delayed or lighter, you should notify your physician.

INSTRUCTIONS FOLLOWING THE TEST

Following the completion of the test you can return to your normal routine. You should avoid douching and intercourse for 2 days. If you develop any fever, chills, severe abdominal pain or heavy vaginal bleeding, you should contact your physician immediately.

ACKNOWLEDGEMENT OF INFORMED CONSENT

I acknowledge that I have read and understand this written material. I understand the purpose, risks and benefits of this procedure. I am aware that there may be other risks and complications not discussed that may occur. I also understand that during the course of the procedure, unforeseen conditions may be revealed requiring the performance of additional procedures. I also understand that technical problems with the instrumentation may prevent the completion of the procedure. I acknowledge that no guarantees or promises have been made to me concerning the results of this procedure or any treatment that may be required as a result of this procedure. I have been given the opportunity to ask questions which have been answered to my satisfaction. I have also considered other options and alternatives. I consent to the performance of the procedure described above by my physician.

_____   _____

Signature of Patient   Signature of Physician

_____

Printed Name

_____

Date of Birth

_____

Date

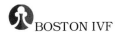BOSTON IVF

CONSENT FORM FOR AN ENDOMETRIAL BIOPSY

An endometrial biopsy is a procedure that involves the removal of endometrial tissue from the uterine cavity for examination. The endometrial biopsy can be performed as part of an infertility evaluation to assess the adequacy of the uterine lining, which is influenced by progesterone levels in the blood. In addition, women who have a history of abnormal bleeding, irregular or absent menstrual periods, or have had a previous endometrial biopsy demonstrating the presence of infection, may benefit from the performance of an endometrial biopsy.

PROCEDURE

The procedure is performed in the office. First, a speculum is placed in the vagina to visualize the cervix. A small plastic catheter is then inserted into the cervical canal and into the uterine cavity. In some cases, it may be necessary to attach an instrument to the cervix to help pass the biopsy catheter into the uterine cavity. After the catheter is inserted, a biopsy of the endometrium is aspirated into the catheter, which is then removed. In most cases, the biopsy is completed within 4–5 minutes. This procedure can be associated with some lower abdominal cramping which will subside after the biopsy is completed. Taking ibuprofen (Motrin®, Advil®) 1 hour before the procedure can minimize cramping. The endometrial biopsy is then sent to the laboratory for an examination by a pathologist. Results of the biopsy are available approximately 1 week after it is performed.

COMPLICATIONS

The complication rate from this procedure is less than 2%. Some of the complications include the following:

1. *Pelvic infection* The performance of this test can result in an infection that could produce lower abdominal pain and fever that develop within a few days following completion of the procedure. A consequence of this infection may be scarred Fallopian tubes and infertility. If an infection develops, hospitalization with IV antibiotics and, potentially, surgery may be indicated.

2. *Exposure of potential pregnancy* A pregnancy test can be performed prior to the performance of the biopsy. However, if the pregnancy is too early the pregnancy test may be negative. If the endometrial biopsy is performed during an early pregnancy there is a possibility that the performance of the biopsy could increase the chance of a miscarriage.

3. ***Uterine perforation*** An uncommon complication of this procedure is perforation of the uterus. If this occurs, the procedure is stopped. Perforation can result in injury to other organs including the intestines, bladder, uterus and blood vessels. Injury to these organs could result in a hospitalization and additional treatment that could include surgery to repair the injury.

INSTRUCTIONS FOLLOWING THE TEST

Following the completion of the test, you can return to your normal routine. You should avoid intercourse and douching for the next 2 days. If you develop any fever, chills, severe abdominal pain or heavy vaginal bleeding, you should contact your physician immediately.

ACKNOWLEDGEMENT OF INFORMED CONSENT

I acknowledge that I have read and understand this written material. I understand the purpose, risks, benefits and alternatives of this procedure. I am aware that there may be other risks and complications not discussed that may occur. I also understand that during the course of the procedure, unforeseen conditions may be revealed requiring the performance of additional procedures. I also understand that technical problems with the instrumentation may prevent the completion of the procedure. I acknowledge that no guarantees or promises have been made to me concerning the results of this procedure or any treatment that may be required as a result of this procedure. I have been given the opportunity to ask questions which have been answered to my satisfaction. I consent to the performance of the procedure described above by my physician.

_____   _____

Signature of Patient   Signature of Physician

_____

Printed Name

_____

Date of Birth

_____

Date

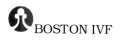BOSTON IVF

CONSENT FORM FOR
TREATMENT WITH OVULATION INDUCTION
MEDICATIONS AND INTRAUTERINE INSEMINATIONS

INTRODUCTION

Ovulation induction medications can help an infertile woman to achieve a pregnancy by stimulating the development of eggs within the ovaries. Ovulation inducing medications are often used in conjunction with intrauterine inseminations with a washed sperm sample. Sometimes intrauterine inseminations are used without any preceding medications. This document explains ovulation inducing medications and intrauterine insemination treatment.

PRETREATMENT RECOMMENDATIONS

During treatment a woman should avoid any activity, behavior and medications that could reduce her chance of conceiving and having a healthy baby. In addition, the recommendations listed below should be followed:

1. A prenatal vitamin should be taken on a daily basis before the treatment is begun. This will reduce the chance that a baby will be born with a neural tube defect (e.g. spina bifida), which is a birth defect that affects the development of the spine.

2. Smoking must be avoided before and during treatment. It is also contraindicated during pregnancy.

3. Recreational drugs are absolutely contraindicated.

4. Ingestion of aspirin or aspirin-like products (e.g. Motrin®, Advil®, Anaprox®, Naprosyn®, Aleve®, etc.) should be avoided during treatment. However, in certain circumstances your doctor may prescribe low dose aspirin (baby aspirin, 81 mg). Tylenol® is safe to take before and during pregnancy.

5. The use of alcohol should be avoided during treatment and after pregnancy is established.

6. The use of all prescription and over-the-counter medications (including herbal remedies) should be discussed with a physician before starting a treatment cycle.

7. HIV (human immunodeficiency virus) screening is strongly recommended for all couples undergoing infertility treatment. HIV is the virus that causes acquired immunodeficiency syndrome (AIDS). A woman infected with HIV

can pass the virus to her unborn child. Please talk to your physician about having this test performed.

DESCRIPTION OF TREATMENT

This treatment involves several steps as outlined below. Patients are not guaranteed success at any or all of these steps. If optimal results are not achieved at any step, it may be recommended that the treatment is stopped and the cycle cancelled.

I. Ovulation induction

The eggs are present in the ovaries in fluid-filled cysts called follicles. During a normal menstrual cycle, usually one mature follicle develops, which results in the ovulation of a single egg. Several hormones, including follicle stimulating hormone (FSH) and luteinizing hormone (LH) influence the growth of the ovarian follicle. These hormones are produced by the pituitary gland, which is located at the base of the brain. FSH is the main hormone that stimulates the growth of the follicle, which produces an estrogen hormone called estradiol. When the follicle is mature, a large amount of LH is released by the pituitary gland. This surge of LH helps to mature the egg and leads to ovulation 36–40 hours after its initiation.

Ovulation induction is a process whereby medications are used to stimulate the ovaries to stimulate egg development and ovulation. The objective of ovulation induction may be to correct an ovulatory problem and/or increase the number of eggs that are released from the ovaries.

A. *Medications*

There are several medications that can be prescribed to stimulate the ovaries. The categories of medications that may be used are discussed below.

1. ***Clomiphene citrate (Serophene®, Clomid®)*** This is an oral, synthetic medication that is taken daily for 5 days. This medication stimulates the release of FSH and LH, which stimulate the development of follicles.

2. ***Gonadotropins*** These are injectable medications commonly prescribed to stimulate the ovaries. Two types of gonadotropins can be prescribed and are discussed below.

    a. ***FSH (Gonal-F®, Follistim®, Fertinex®)*** These medications contain only FSH and are administered on a daily basis by subcutaneous injection.

b. *Human menopausal gonadotropins (Pergonal®, Humegon®, Repronex®)* These medications contain FSH and LH, and are administered on a daily basis by intramuscular or subcutaneous injection.

3. *GnRH agonist (Lupron®, Synarel®)* These synthetic hormones are administered by subcutaneous injection (Lupron) or an intranasal spray (Synarel). The administration of a GnRH agonist initially causes release of FSH and LH from the pituitary gland. However, with continued administration there is a temporary depletion of FSH and LH, which suppresses a LH surge thereby preventing ovulation. GnRH agonists are administered in conjunction with gonadotropins.

4. *GnRH antagonist (Cetrotide®, Antagon®)* GnRH antagonists are medications that reversibly bind to GnRH receptors in the pituitary gland and prevent release of FSH and LH. GnRH antagonists are administered in combination with gonadotropins. The major benefit of a GnRH antagonist is that it suppresses a LH surge thereby preventing ovulation.

5. *Human chorionic gonadotropin (hCG) (Profasi®, Ovidrel®, Pregnyl®, Novarel®)* This medication contains the pregnancy hormone, hCG, which functions similarly to LH. During the medical treatment when the follicles have reached a stage of maturity the administration of hCG will cause ovulation to occur.

Note: Many of the medications that are used are administered by an injection. The patient or another person can be instructed to give these injections.

B. *Side-effects*

The use of the above-listed medications can cause side-effects such as nausea, vomiting, hot flashes, headaches, mood swings, visual symptoms, memory difficulties, joint problems, weight gain and weight loss, all of which are temporary. Allergic reactions, although rare, are also possible. Other possible side-effects include the following:

1. *Ovarian hyperstimulation* After ovulation, the collapsed ovarian follicles can fill up with fluid and form cysts. The formation of cysts will result in ovarian enlargement and can lead to lower abdominal discomfort, bloating and distention. These symptoms generally occur within 2 weeks after ovulation. The symptoms usually resolve within 1–2 weeks without intervention. If ovarian hyperstimulation occurs your physician may recommend a period of reduced activity and bed rest. Pregnancy can worsen the symptoms of ovarian

hyperstimulation. Severe ovarian hyperstimulation is characterized by the development of large ovarian cysts and fluid in the abdominal and, sometimes, chest cavities. Symptoms of severe ovarian hyperstimulation include abdominal distention and bloating along with weight gain, shortness of breath, nausea, vomiting and decreased urine output. Approximately 1–2% of women will develop severe ovarian hyperstimulation and may need to be admitted to the hospital for observation and treatment. Rare, but serious consequences of severe ovarian hyperstimulation include formation of blood clots that can lead to a stroke, kidney damage and possibly death. Every woman who takes these medications can develop ovarian hyperstimulation but the chance is higher in a woman with a high blood estradiol level and a large number of ovarian follicles. In some cases when the estradiol level is significantly elevated, the cycle may be cancelled or the eggs will be retrieved and any embryos that result will be frozen.

2. *Ovarian torsion (twisting)* In less than 1% of cases, a fluid-filled cyst(s) in the ovary can cause the ovary to twist on itself. This can decrease the blood supply to the ovary and result in significant lower abdominal pain. Surgery may be required to untwist or possibly remove the ovary.

3. *Ovarian cancer* In the general population, every woman has a 1 in 70 chance of developing ovarian cancer during her lifetime. Studies have shown that infertile women have a higher chance of developing ovarian cancer than fertile women. Controversial data exist that associate the use of ovulation induction drugs (e.g. clomiphene citrate, gonadotropins) with an increased risk of ovarian cancer. However, presently a cause and effect relationship has not been clearly established.

C. *Monitoring*

During the ovulation induction phase of treatment, monitoring of follicular development is performed with a urinary ovulation predictor kit or periodic blood hormone tests and vaginal ultrasound exams. Monitoring helps the physician to determine the appropriate dose of medication and the timing of ovulation. Vaginal ultrasound examinations are usually painless and generally considered to be safe. However, the possibility of harm cannot be excluded. Blood drawing may be associated with mild discomfort and, possibly, bruising, bleeding, infection or scarring at the needle sites. The need for repeated ultrasound examinations and blood drawing on a frequent basis requires the woman's presence in the vicinity of her physician's office.

II. Intrauterine insemination

Around the time of ovulation, a woman receiving ovulation inducing medications will be instructed to either have intercourse or an intrauterine insemination (IUI) with a washed sperm sample. On the day of the IUI treatment, the male partner will be asked to produce a semen specimen at the Center. The semen sample can be produced at home as long as it can be brought into the Center within 1 hour after it is produced. It is important that the semen sample is kept at body temperature during transport. The semen sample will then be washed and prepared. In some cases, the woman (or couple) may elect to use a donor sperm sample.

To perform an IUI a speculum is placed in the vagina and the cervix is visualized. Sperm are loaded into a catheter, which is inserted through the cervical canal and into the uterine cavity. Following the insemination, normal activity can be resumed. Because a catheter is inserted into the uterine cavity during the insemination treatment, there is always the risk of a pelvic infection following the treatment. Symptoms of an infection include fever, vaginal bleeding, chills and abdominal pain. If any of these symptoms occur you should contact your physician. In rare cases, hospitalization with intravenous antibiotics and/or surgery (to remove ovaries, Fallopian tubes, or the uterus) may be necessary. As a result fertility may be impaired in some cases.

Non-medicated IUI treatment is less commonly used than the medicated approach. If a woman has regular menstrual cycles, a non-medicated cycle may be considered. With this approach, the development of the single follicle is monitored with an ovulation predictor kit or blood tests and ultrasound examinations. When the follicle is mature and ovulation is imminent, the IUI treatment will be planned. In contrast to the medicated approach, there is a lower chance of pregnancy because only one egg is released for possible fertilization.

III. Treatment following ovulation

Fourteen days after ovulation has occurred, a blood pregnancy can be performed. If this test is found to be positive, a repeat pregnancy test may be done 2–3 days later. If the test results are encouraging, a vaginal ultrasound will be done approximately 4 weeks after the treatments to determine the status of the pregnancy. Because of the potential for complications following ovulation induction, the woman should have access to medical care up to the time of the pregnancy test and beyond if pregnancy is established. If travel is absolutely necessary, it should be discussed with a physician.

TREATMENT OUTCOMES

The success (the delivery of a live born infant) following a cycle of treatment with the administration of ovulation induction medications is 5–20% per cycle. The development of a pregnancy following this treatment is dependent on many factors, some of which include: the age of the woman, the infertility diagnosis, the number of previous cycles of treatment, the number of follicles that develop, and the quality of the sperm.

An overview of some of the more common risks of pregnancy are discussed below:

Miscarriage

The risk of miscarriage in the general population is 15–20%. The risk of miscarriage increases with the age of the woman and for women over 40 years of age, the risk may exceed 50%. Studies have shown either no increase or a slight increase in the risk of miscarriage in women who conceive with this treatment. Most miscarriages are associated with lower abdominal cramping and bleeding, but do not necessarily require treatment. In some cases, however, complete removal of the pregnancy tissue must be accomplished by a surgical procedure called a dilatation and curettage (D&C). This procedure is usually performed under anesthesia in the operating room and involves placing a suction tube into the uterine cavity to remove the pregnancy tissue.

Tubal (ectopic) pregnancy

An ectopic pregnancy may develop as a result of this treatment. The majority of ectopic pregnancies are present in the Fallopian tube. The chance of tubal pregnancy is greater in a woman with damaged tubes. If a woman has a tubal pregnancy, she may need surgical treatment, which may involve the removal of the involved tube. Medical treatment with methotrexate may be an option in selected cases.

Multiple pregnancy

The administration of ovulation induction medications can result in the ovulation of more than one egg, which increases the chance of a multiple pregnancy. The chance of multiple pregnancy ranges from 8 to 25%, which is in part dependent on the medication that is used. For instance, following clomiphene citrate treatment the multiple pregnancy rate ranges between 8 and 12%. When the injectable medications are used (gonadotropins) the multiple pregnancy rate is between 20 and 25%. Of the multiple pregnancies, approximately 80% are twins and the remainder (20%) are triplets and quadruplets. The chance of quadruplets is less than 2% of all pregnancies. Rarely, more than quadruplets can result. All multiple pregnancies are associated with an increased risk of most complications of pregnancy including, but not limited to, miscarriage, toxemia, congenital anomalies, gestational diabetes in the mother and premature labor and birth. Premature birth is the single greatest cause of death or disability in newborn infants. In contrast to a single intrauterine pregnancy, a multiple pregnancy may pose increased emotional and financial hardship.

If a multiple pregnancy develops, the couple may consider being referred to a specialist who can perform a multifetal reduction procedure. This procedure, which is performed at approximately 3 months of pregnancy, is carried out to reduce the number of pregnancy sacs to a lower and safer number. Although this procedure is successful 90–95% of the time, a complete miscarriage may result.

Other risks

Most infants who have been born following fertility treatment are normal. The rate of congenital abnormalities (birth defects) in the general population is 2–3% and is not different in babies conceived following this treatment. It is important to be aware that genetic abnormalities, structural abnormalities, mental retardation and other abnormalities may occur following this treatment or as they do in pregnancies conceived naturally.

Psychological risks

Undergoing infertility treatment can be psychologically stressful. Anxiety and disappointment may occur at any point during and after treatment. Significant commitment of time and, at times, finances may be required. All couples are encouraged to meet with a counselor. There are many complex, and sometimes unknown, factors which may prevent the establishment of pregnancy. Known factors, which may prevent the establishment of pregnancy, include, but are not limited to, the following:

1. The ovaries may not respond to the medications or the ovarian follicles may not develop during the treatment.

2. The ovaries may over respond to the medication and the cycle may be cancelled because of the increased risk of ovarian hyperstimulation and/or multiple pregnancy.

3. The male partner may be unable to ejaculate or the semen sample may be of poor quality.

4. The passage of the catheter into the uterus may be technically difficult or impossible.

5. Even if the insemination is successfully performed, pregnancy may not result.

6. If a pregnancy is established, it may not develop normally.

7. Equipment failure, infection, technical problems, human errors and/or other unforeseen factors may result in loss or damage to the semen sample.

ACKNOWLEDGEMENT OF INFORMED CONSENT AND AUTHORIZATION

We acknowledge that we, the undersigned, are voluntarily undergoing, treatment in order to conceive a child through this treatment and that we acknowledge our natural parentage of any child born through this technique.

We acknowledge that we have read and fully understand this written material, we have considered treatment alternatives, and all of my questions concerning the treatment have been fully answered to my satisfaction.

By consenting to treatment we accept the responsibilities, conditions and risks involved as set out in this document and as explained by the staff. In addition, we consent to the techniques and procedures used in this treatment as described in this document and as explained by the staff.

We acknowledge and agree that our acceptance into treatment and continued participation is within the sole discretion of my physician.

We understand that should these cycles be unsuccessful, it may be determined that further treatment may not be indicated. We also understand that we are financially responsible for any medical expenses that are not covered by the insurance policy.

We understand that medical information concerning my treatment may be analyzed and could be used in a publication.

We, the undersigned, consent to undergo this treatment. We have read this document, understand the purpose, risks and benefits of this procedure, and we have been given the opportunity to ask questions, which have been answered to our satisfaction by our physician and the staff.

_____   _____   _____
Signature of Female   Signature of Male   Signature of Physician

_____   _____   _____
Printed Name   Printed Name   Date

_____   _____
Date of Birth   Date of Birth

_____   _____
Date   Date

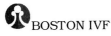BOSTON IVF

CONSENT FORM FOR
METHOTREXATE TREATMENT

INTRODUCTION

When a normal pregnancy is established, the fertilized egg or the embryo implants in the uterine cavity. However, sometimes the embryo implants outside of the uterine cavity. This situation is referred to as an ectopic pregnancy and cannot lead to a normal pregnancy. The vast majority of ectopic pregnancies (> 95%) occur in the Fallopian tube but an ectopic pregnancy can also implant in the cervix, ovary or abdominal cavity. The major concern with an ectopic pregnancy is that it can rupture through the Fallopian tube and result in internal bleeding.

In the past, the diagnosis of tubal pregnancy was made when the pregnancy was more advanced and surgical removal of the tube was usually necessary. With the development of vaginal ultrasound and a sensitive pregnancy test, the diagnosis of an ectopic pregnancy can be made earlier. When the diagnosis is made at an earlier stage, there is a greater likelihood that the ectopic pregnancy can be removed surgically and the Fallopian tube can be conserved.

Methotrexate administration is available as an alternative to surgery. This medication stops rapidly dividing cells from multiplying (pregnancy tissue grows in this fashion). Methotrexate is a chemotherapy drug, which has been used to treat women with molar pregnancies. Molar pregnancies are non-viable intrauterine pregnancies that are made up of very aggressive placental tissue that can grow into the wall of the uterus. Several studies have demonstrated that properly selected patients with ectopic pregnancies can be successfully treated with methotrexate.

INDICATIONS FOR METHOTREXATE

Methotrexate treatment has several applications in the treatment of ectopic pregnancy, which are discussed below.

1. ***Persistent ectopic pregnancy following conservative surgery*** If the diagnosis is made early, an ectopic pregnancy can be removed from the Fallopian tube by a surgical procedure called laparoscopy. This procedure is performed under general anesthesia and involves the placement of a telescope-like instrument and other instruments through small incisions in the abdomen. A small incision is made in the tube over the ectopic pregnancy and the pregnancy tissue is removed. However, not all of the tissue can be removed and some remains in the tube. In the majority of cases, the remaining pregnancy tissue

goes away on its own but in other cases the tissue can remain in the tube and continue to grow. Following conservative surgery, periodic blood samples are taken to follow the level of the pregnancy hormone, human chorionic gonadotropin (hCG). As long as the hCG level decreases no intervention is necessary. However, if the hCG levels plateau or increase, additional treatment is indicated. Treatment options include repeat laparoscopy with possible removal of the Fallopian tube or medical treatment with methotrexate.

2. *An ectopic pregnancy in a location that is not amenable to conservative surgery* If the ectopic pregnancy is located in the cervix, the ovary or in the portion of the tube that is located in the uterine wall, surgical removal may be difficult and potentially complicated. Treatment with methotrexate is another alternative.

3. *A woman who is a poor operative risk* Medical treatment can be considered for the woman who is at greater risk for surgical or anesthetic complications.

4. *A presumed ectopic pregnancy* Some women who achieve pregnancy have slowly rising levels of pregnancy hormone. In this situation, there is no chance for a viable pregnancy. This occurrence can be the result of a failed intrauterine pregnancy or an ectopic pregnancy. Another presentation of an ectopic pregnancy is when an ultrasound exam fails to document an intrauterine pregnancy at 6 weeks of pregnancy and/or when the hCG titer has reached 2000 mIU/ml. In these situations there are several alternatives:

    a. *Performance of a D&C* This procedure involves placing an instrument into the uterine cavity to remove the pregnancy tissue. This surgery is performed under anesthesia. A pathologist can examine the tissue and if pregnancy tissue is identified, the presence of a failed intrauterine pregnancy is confirmed and no further treatment is indicated. Alternatively, if the pathologist fails to identify pregnancy tissue, then this raises further suspicion of an ectopic pregnancy. If this occurs, there are two options – medical treatment with methotrexate or surgical treatment by laparoscopy.

    b. *Methotrexate treatment* The other option is to not undergo a D&C and be treated with methotrexate initially. A single intramuscular injection will be administered and you will be asked to return for weekly blood work to have the pregnancy hormone level assessed. If the level decreases, then simple observation is indicated. Alternatively, if the level increases or plateaus a second injection of methotrexate or surgery may be indicated.

5. **Confirmed ectopic pregnancy** If an ultrasound exam confirms the presence of a gestational sac (evidence of an early pregnancy) outside of the uterine cavity then the diagnosis of an ectopic pregnancy is established. In this situation there are two options:

   a. **Laparoscopy** This is an outpatient surgical procedure that is performed under general anesthesia. The procedure involves the placement of a telescopic instrument through a small incision into the abdominal cavity, allowing visualization of the pelvic organs. When the ectopic pregnancy is localized in the tube then a small incision in the tube to remove the pregnancy tissue. During the postoperative period pregnancy hormone levels will be followed until they are negative. If at the time of the laparoscopy there is significant damage to the tube then partial or complete removal of the tube may be indicated. At the time of surgery the other tube will be examined to determine its condition.

   b. **Methotrexate treatment** This treatment is reviewed below.

METHOTREXATE TREATMENT

If you elect to proceed with methotrexate treatment, the first step is to obtain a routine blood work-up. If it is determined that you are a candidate for this treatment, the methotrexate will be administered by an intramuscular injection. Side-effects may occur but do not usually appear until 2–7 days after administration. Side-effects include nausea, vomiting, abdominal pain and loss of appetite. Sores or ulcers of the mouth, tongue, vagina and bowel occur rarely, are usually mild and resolve over a short period of time. Rarely, methotrexate can lower the white blood and platelet counts. Other very uncommon side-effects include hair loss, skin rash, dizziness and liver dysfunction. Because of the potential liver toxicity it is important that you do not consume any alcohol while taking this medication.

A pregnancy blood level (hCG) will be determined at weekly intervals. If the level is dropping, then the pregnancy hormone level will be followed periodically until it reaches zero. It can take up to 4–5 weeks or sometimes longer after the injection of methotrexate before the pregnancy hormone level reaches zero. If the pregnancy hormone level plateaus or increases, then either another injection can be administered or surgery can be performed.

It is important to remember that even though you have received methotrexate, tubal rupture can still occur and emergency surgery may be required. Therefore, you should contact your doctor immediately if you develop abdominal pain.

Even though your tubal pregnancy totally resolves on methotrexate treatment, scarring may occur in your tube as a result of the tubal pregnancy as it can following surgical treatment. This could predispose you to a tubal pregnancy in the future and/or subsequent infertility. Your chances of conceiving after medical therapy with methotrexate are the same as after surgery. There is no increased risk of congenital anomalies in babies born to women who have taken methotrexate in the past.

It is important that during and up to 2 weeks after receiving methotrexate you should not drink any alcohol or take aspirin or aspirin-like compounds (Advil®, Motrin®, etc.), folic acid or vitamins containing folic acid. You should also avoid excess exposure to sun or use of sunlamps for 4 weeks following methotrexate therapy because your skin may be more sensitive to sunlight than usual and you can burn excessively. You should also avoid intercourse until resolution.

ACKNOWLEDGEMENT OF INFORMED CONSENT

I acknowledge that I have read and understand this written material. I understand the purpose, risks and benefits of methotrexate treatment. I am aware that there may be other risks and complications of the treatment not discussed that may occur. I also understand that during the course of the procedure, unforeseen conditions may be revealed requiring the performance of additional procedures. I acknowledge that no guarantees or promises have been made to me concerning the results of this treatment or any treatment that may be required as a result of this procedure. I have been given the opportunity to ask questions which have been answered to my satisfaction. I have also considered other options and alternatives. I consent to methotrexate administration.

_____   _____

Signature of Patient   Signature of Physician

_____

Printed Name

_____

Date of Birth

_____

Date

11.

Counseling

Infertility is a medical problem that has a significant psychological component. The infertile woman can experience feelings of anxiety, guilt, inadequacy, poor self-esteem and overt depression. For many it is hard to understand how infertility can be so emotionally taxing. It is not a serious medical condition and surely no one has ever died from the diagnosis. However, the explanation is simple – reproduction and nurturing offspring is one of the most significant life experiences. Taking this into consideration it is understandable how infertility produces stress. In fact, the stress felt by the infertile patient is comparable in magnitude to the stress experienced when a life-threatening condition such as cancer or heart disease is diagnosed. In addition to the effects on the individual, the stress can put strain on a marriage and impact relationships with family and friends. All of these reactions can be further amplified by the disappointment of failed treatment. Individuals cope with these feelings in different ways depending on their personality and life experiences. Few situations in life can be as challenging, demanding and overwhelming.

Much of the psychological reaction experienced by the infertile couple stems from the lack of control. As we venture through life we are taught that if we work hard and follow the rules we will be rewarded with success. This is not always true when it comes to fertility. This is in part because the human reproductive system is inefficient. It is important that this is conveyed to couples so they do not proceed with unrealistic expectations. In the best of circumstances, a *fertile* couple has only a 15–20% chance of achieving a pregnancy during any month. Further, if pregnancy is established, there is a 20–30% chance of a miscarriage. Even when the problem has been corrected and an optimal situation is created, success rates following infertility treatment only range between 10 and 40% per cycle. In many instances, we do not have a good explanation for the couple when the treatment fails, which only adds to the stress and bewilderment of the process. Another situation that can be stressful is when the couple is diagnosed with unexplained infertility. Approximately 25% of infertile couples have unexplained infertility despite a complete evaluation.

From the physician's perspective the diagnosis of unexplained infertility is not of concern because the couple has an excellent chance of achieving pregnancy with treatment. However, for the couple it can be quite distressing because they are in search of answers.

It is important at the initial consultation that the psychological reaction the couple is experiencing is assessed. Virtually every infertile couple that presents is emotionally stressed to some degree. Patients should be told that their reactions and feelings are normal. Counseling and support should be made available to all couples. In some cases, the psychological symptoms are significant enough to warrant a referral to a mental health professional before an evaluation or treatment is begun.

DOES STRESS CAUSE INFERTILITY?

It is not disputed that infertility can lead to stress, but controversy exists as to whether stress can lead to infertility. The stress response results in hormonal and physiological changes that could theoretically alter reproductive function in both men and women. We have all heard stories about a couple who achieves pregnancy after a relaxing vacation or an infertile woman who achieves pregnancy on her own after a successful adoption. However, these are random events and there are no conclusive studies in the literature that establish stress as a cause of infertility. Some have advocated the use of relaxation techniques to help reduce the stress. Relaxation techniques include imagery, breath techniques, yoga, meditation and prayer. The benefits of these techniques have been confirmed in many realms of medicine. While the benefits on fertility have not been proven, practicing these techniques helps the infertile couples deal better with the stress by putting them back into control.

WHO CAN BENEFIT FROM COUNSELING?

Every couple should be made aware that counseling is available and assessable. Individuals with signs or symptoms of depression or other psychopathology should be referred for counseling and a psychological assessment. Any couple who is considering whether to stop treatment or is exploring other options including gamete donation, adoption, or gestational carrier treatment would benefit from counseling. Another patient who would benefit from counseling is one who has experienced a pregnancy loss. It is well documented in the literature that many women experience a grief reaction following a pregnancy loss.

WHERE CAN COUPLES GET HELP?

Mental health professionals including social workers, psychologists and psychiatrists are trained to evaluate and treat couples who are in crisis. Because of the complexities of infertility and the treatment options that are available, couples would benefit most from a referral to a professional with experience in the field of infertility. RESOLVE and the American Infertility Association are valuable resources for infertile couples to seek out qualified mental health professionals.

> ➢ **RESOLVE**
> 1310 Broadway
> Somerville, MA 02144–1731
> Phone: (617)–623–1156
> *www.resolve.org*

> ➢ **American Infertility Association**
> 666 Fifth Avenue, Suite 278
> New York, NY 10103
> Phone: (718)–621–5083
> *www.americaninfertility.org*

HOW DOES A COUPLE LEARN MORE ABOUT ADOPTION?

The first step is to follow up with a mental health professional to talk about the emotional and practical issues about the process. There are many different variations of the adoption process including anonymous and identified adoption; national and international opportunities also exist. The couple can be referred to the following resources for additional information and learn more about the process:

> ➢ **National Council for Adoption**
> 1930 17th Street NW
> Washington, DC 20009–6207
> Phone: (202)–328–1200
> Fax: (202)–332–0935
> e-mail: *ncfa@ncfa-usa.org*
> *www.ncfa-usa.org/*

➢ **National Adoption Information Clearing House**
330 C Street, SW
Washington, DC 20447
Phone: (703)–352–3488 or (888)–251–0075
Fax: (703)–385–3206
e-mail: *naic@calib.com*
www.calib.com/naic

➢ **RESOLVE**
1310 Broadway
Somerville, MA 02144–1731
Phone: (617)–623–1156
www.resolve.org

➢ **American Infertility Association**
666 Fifth Avenue, Suite 278
New York, NY 10103
Phone: (718)–621–5083
www.americaninfertility.org

12.

Educational resources

BOSTON IVF

- *Web site – **www.bostonivf.com***
- Our web site provides a broad overview of infertility treatments and links to other important sites

SERONO LABORATORIES

100 Longwater Circle
Norwell, MA 02061

- Patient education booklets are available and are ***free*** of charge
- Contact your local Serono sales representative

Topics

- ➤ Assisted reproductive technologies
- ➤ Infertility: the emotional roller coaster
- ➤ Infertility over 35
- ➤ Insights into infertility
- ➤ Infertility: the male factor
- ➤ Pathways to parenthood

ORGANON INC.

575 Pleasant Ave.
West Orange, NJ 07052

- Patient education booklets are available and ***free*** of charge
- Contact your local Organon sales representative

Topics

➢ Assisted reproductive technologies
➢ Uterine insemination
➢ Ovulation induction
➢ Polycystic ovaries
➢ Treatment guide

FERRING PHARMACEUTICALS

120 White Plains Rd Suite 400
Tarrytown, NY 10591

- This drug company has put together a compilation of one-page handouts that can be given to the patient regarding the evaluation, causes of infertility and treatment
- Call your local Ferring representative

AMERICAN SOCIETY FOR REPRODUCTIVE MEDICINE (ASRM)

1209 Montogomery Highway
Birmingham, ALA 35216

- 1–205–978–5000
- *Web site – **www.asrm.org***
- This organization has been a leader in the field of reproductive medicine and publishes a patient education series of booklets that can be purchased for about $1.00 for each copy

Topics

➢ Adoption
➢ Age and fertility
➢ Birth defects of the female reproductive system
➢ Donor insemination
➢ Early menopause
➢ Endometriosis
➢ Fertility after cancer treatment
➢ Hirsutism and the polycystic ovarian disease syndrome
➢ Husband insemination
➢ Infertility – an overview
➢ Infertility – coping and decision making
➢ IVF & GIFT: a guide to the assisted reproductive technologies
➢ Laparoscopy and hysteroscopy
➢ Ovulation drugs
➢ Pregnancy after infertility

➢ Third party reproduction
(Donor eggs, donor sperm
donor embryos and surrogacy)

➢ Tubal factor infertility

➢ Unexplained infertility

RESOLVE

National Office:

1310 Broadway
Somerville, MA 02144–1731

- Phone: 1–617–623–1156
- *Web site – **www.resolve.org***
- RESOLVE is a nationwide patient advocacy group that was first established in Massachusetts. They are an invaluable resource for patients and health-care providers. The services they provide are diverse including: support groups, physician referrals, publications addressing infertility, advocacy network and the publication of a quarterly newsletter

AMERICAN INFERTILITY ASSOCIATION (AIA)

666 Fifth Avenue, Suite 278
New York, NY 10103

- Phone: 1–718–621–5083
- *Web site – **www.americaninfertility.org***
- The AIA is a patient advocacy group that services the New England area. They are a resource for infertile couples and practitioners. They provide a wide array of services including support groups, educational resources, per support network, a newsletter and an informative web site

13.

Insurance and coding issues

Before any medical services are provided, it is essential that the patient's insurance coverage be investigated. This will help to insure that any services that are rendered will be properly reimbursed and will eliminate the chance that the patient will receive any unexpected bills. Some of the important insurance issues regarding infertility services are discussed below. In addition, guidelines for current procedural terminology coding for infertility services are presented.

WHEN SHOULD THERE BE AN INVESTIGATION OF THE INSURANCE COVERAGE?

At the initial consultation, when the couple is to begin a medical evaluation, it is time to do an insurance evaluation as well. Documentation of medical insurance coverage for both partners should be reviewed. An updated insurance card should be copied and placed in the patient's chart. Verification of infertility benefits should be obtained by contacting the insurance company or reviewing the insurance policy. The extent and the limitations of coverage should also be determined. If there are any restrictions in the insurance coverage, it is important that this is discussed with the couple before they undergo any medical services. If the couple wants to challenge the limitations of their insurance coverage then they have recourse. The first option is that the couple can present their case in front of the appeals board of the insurance company. The other option is that the couple can contact the state insurance commissioner, who acts on behalf of consumers. Couples who do not have any insurance benefits should be encouraged to look for other insurance plans that may provide coverage for infertility services.

WHAT STATES HAVE MANDATED INFERTILITY BENEFITS?

Infertility treatment has been viewed as elective and many insurance companies have chosen not to pay for it. In 1987, Massachusetts passed a bill that defined infertility as a medical diagnosis and therefore mandated insurance companies in the state to pay for infertility treatment. Other states have followed suit including: Arkansas, California, Connecticut, Hawaii, Illinois, Maryland, Montana, New Jersey, New York, Ohio, Rhode Island, Texas and West Virginia. Detailed state-specific information can be obtained by visiting the web site of the American Society for Reproductive Medicine (*www.asrm.org*). If you reside in a state that does not have mandated insurance benefits for infertility, you can contact RESOLVE, a patient advocacy organization (see Chapter 12) to find out if there is any pending legislation. Even if your state does have mandated benefits, restrictions can still exist regarding the extent and types of infertility treatment that are covered. In addition, within mandated states, privately insured companies often can eliminate infertility services as a covered benefit.

CODING AND BILLING ISSUES

After medical services have been provided, the next step is to get reimbursed from the insurance company in an expeditious fashion. This is achieved by Complete Procedure Terminology (CPT) coding that is in agreement with the diagnostic codes that are submitted. Accurate CPT coding helps to maximize reimbursements and to avoid costly audits by insurance companies. A complete review of CPT coding is beyond the scope of this handbook. CPT coding is a complicated process that is constantly changing. All physicians need to be educated and well versed on the intricacies of the coding process. The American Medical Association (AMA) and the American College of Obstetrics and Gynecology (ACOG) publish excellent reference manuals that are updated on an annual basis and should be reviewed. The coding for specific procedures regarding infertility treatments is discussed below.

Evaluation and management (E/M) CPT codes

The E/M codes are applied to office visits. The E/M services include new patient office visits (CPT codes 99241–99245, 99201–99205) and repeat visits (CPT codes 99211–99215). A new patient is one that has not been seen in consultation by the treating physician or by another physician in his/her group in the past 3 years. There are two choices for coding after a new patient office visit:

(1) If a physician or other appropriate authority has requested an opinion regarding the evaluation and treatment of a particular medical problem then the consultation CPT codes are used (99241–99245). After the consultation a

letter needs to be sent to the referring physician. These consultation codes can only be used once. After a physician has assumed care of the patient for any follow-up consultations, the repeat visit codes should be used (99211–99215).

(2) If a new patient has not been referred by another physician the CPT codes 99201–99205 should be used.

The key components of the E/M codes include the history, physical examination, medical decision-making, counseling, coordination of care, nature of presenting problem and time. The first three components of this list (history, physical examination and medical decision-making) are the key components that determine the level of coding.

(1) For the new patient visits (99241–99245, 99201–99205) all three key components need to be performed and documented.

(2) For repeat visits (99211–99215) two out the three key components should be performed and documented.

However, in many cases at the time of the office visit the majority of the physician's time is spent counseling the couple and the key components necessary for the coding are not performed. In these situations, the time spent can be the controlling factor to determine the level of the coding but it needs to be documented in the chart. An excerpt from the AMA CPT coding manual addresses this issue:

> 'In the case when counseling and/or coordination of care dominates (more than 50%) the physician/patient encounter (face-to-face time in the office or other outpatient setting or floor/unit time in the hospital), then time may be considered the key or controlling factor to qualify for a particular level of E/M services. The extent of counseling and/or coordination of care must be documented in the medical record.'

The amount of face-to-face time (in minutes) needed to determine the level of coding is described in the AMA CPT handbook and is as follows:

99241 15'	99201 10'	99211 5'
99242 30'	99202 20'	99212 10'
99243 40'	99203 30'	99213 15'
99244 60'	99204 45'	99214 25'
99245 80'	99205 60'	99215 40'

Coding for specific office procedures

The CPT codes that can be used for various office procedures are listed below. If a consultation takes place either before or after the procedure is performed then the appropriate E/M code should be selected but a modifier (–25) must be added. Time spent discussing the procedure or reviewing the consent with the patient is felt to be inclusive in the code of the procedure and should not be billed separately.

A. Endometrial biopsy[†]

    81025 – urine pregnancy testing
    58100 – performance of endometrial biopsy
    99070 – supplies

B. Hysterosalpingogram[†]

    81025 – urine pregnancy testing
    58340 – induction of dye

C. Sonohysterogram[†]

    81025 – urine pregnancy testing
    76830 – ultrasound exam of uterus/ovaries
    76831 – hysterosonography
    58340 – induction of saline
    99070 – supplies

D. Insemination treatments

    Intracervical (donor insemination) – 58321
    Intrauterine insemination
        – sperm washing – 58323
        – limited semen analysis – 89310
        – performance of the insemination – 58322

E. Injections (i.e. hCG, methotrexate) – 90782

[†]In some cases a paracervical block (CPT code – 64435) and/or a cervical dilation (CPT code – 57800) are necessary to complete these procedures. If so, these procedure codes should be submitted for reimbursement.

Billing for surgical procedures

To maximize reimbursement for surgical procedures the CPT codes should be submitted along with supporting diagnostic codes. There are several important points concerning billing for surgical procedures, which are described below. It is important that the physician work with the billing personnel to make sure the coding is done correctly.

Relative value units (RVU)

Insurance companies base reimbursement for a procedure on the number of RVU. The Medicare Resource Based Relative Value Scale (RBRVS) was implemented in 1992 as a means to determine physician reimbursement for services on Medicare patients but all insurance companies have adopted it as well. The system is updated every 5 years and the next update is due in January 2002. The RVU is a measure of the time and intensity of the procedure that is performed. For instance, a diagnostic hysteroscopy has 5.76 RVU while a hysteroscopic resection of a uterine septum has 11.62 RVU. The number of RVU for a procedure is directly related to the level of reimbursement. If multiple procedures are performed it is important that the primary procedue (with the most RVU) is listed first then all secondary procedures are listed in descending order of decreasing RVU with a modifier 51. Generally the primary procedure is reimbursed at 100%, then the secondary procedures are reimbursed at a lower percentage.

Bundling

Bundling is a process whereby the CPT codes of multiple procedures are combined into one. For example a patient who underwent a hysteroscopy with a polypectomy would be assigned the CPT code 58558. During the procedure a cervical dilation (57800), a diagnostic hysteroscopy (58120) and a D&C (58120) were performed. All of these procedures have separate CPT codes. However, these procedures cannot be separately billed because the CPT code for the operative hysteroscopy (58558) is bundled and includes these procedures.

Global reimbursement

Payment for a surgical service is a global type reimbursement that covers a period of time prior to and following the surgery. The global payment may include the time spent doing the preoperative history and physical examination. Following the surgery, any routine follow-up care during the postoperative period (ranging from 0–90 days depending on the procedure) may also be included in the global period. The definition of the global period can vary and the insurance company should be contacted to determine their definition.

Using modifiers

Modifiers are ways to redefine a surgical procedure or an evaluation and management code under special circumstances. The use of modifiers is necessary to be reimbursed for the extent of the services provided. The ACOG and the AMA coding manuals provide a description of these modifiers. There are several situations that make it necessary to use modifiers to get reimbursed. Examples of some of these situations are as follows:

- A consultation with the patient occurs on the same day of an office procedure (i.e. endometrial biopsy). *(Modifier –25)*
- An office visit takes place and a decision is made to perform the surgery that same day. *(Modifier –57)*
- The surgical procedure is more complicated and takes additional time. *(Modifier –22)*
- An open laparoscopy is performed. *(Modifier –22)*
- At the time of surgery bilateral procedures are performed on the ovaries (or tubes). *(Modifier –50)*
- Multiple surgeries are performed on the same day. *(Modifier –51)*
- A repeat procedure is performed by the same physician within the global period. *(Modifier –76)*
- A surgical assistant is used when a resident is unavailable. *(Modifier –80/82)*
- A procedure is started but aborted. *(Modifier –53)*

ICD–9–CM diagnostic codes

The CPT code for any E/M or procedure must be accompanied by a compatible diagnosis. The current system in use is the *International Classification of Diseases, Ninth Revision, Clinical Modification (ICD–9–CM)*. Some of the commonly used diagnostic codes for infertility services are presented below:

Infertility		Endocrine		Other	
Anovulation	628.0	Hyperprolactinemia	253.1	Pelvic adhesions	614.6
Cervical factor	628.4	Hyperandrogenism	256.1	Cervical stenosis	622.4
Male factor		Premature ovarian		Endometriosis	617.3
azoospermia	606.0	failure	256.3	Endometrioma	617.1
oligospermia	606.1	Anovulation	628.0	Leiomyoma	218.9
Tubal blockage	628.2	Amenorrhea	626		
Unexplained	628.9				
Non-specified	628.8				

Available resources for coding issues

(1) Publications by the American Medical Association (*www.ama-asn.org/catalog*).
Call 1–800–621–8335 to order.

(2) *International Classifications of Diseases, 9th Revision; Clinical Modification (ICD9 • CM), 5th edition;* published by Medicode, Inc. 5225 Wiley Way, Suite 500, Salt Lake City, UT 84116. 1–800–536–1000.

(3) American College of Obstetricians and Gynecologists (ACOG) resources:
CPT Coding in Obstetrics and Gynecology, 2000 edition.
ACOG web site (*www.acog.com*).
Departmental web site – *Coding and Nomenclature.*

14.

Quick reference

Basic Infertility Evaluation
➢ CD 3-FSH, estradiol
➢ Hysterosalpingogram
➢ Semen analysis
➢ Preconceptional blood work
• TSH
• CBC
• Blood type & screen
• RPR
• Antibody screens for:
– Rubella
– Varicella
– Hepatitis
– HIV
• Genetic screening (if indicated)
➢ Laparoscopy (optional)

Interpretation of cycle day 3 hormone levels

Follicle Level (mIu/ml)	Estradiol Level (pg/ml)	Ovarian Reserve
> 10	< 70	↓
> 10	> 70	↓
2–10	> 70	↓
2–10	< 70	normal

Clomiphene citrate challenge test
1. Cycle day 3 – FSH + estradiol levels
2. Clomiphene citrate 100 mg cycle days 5–9
3. Cycle day 10 – FSH level
Interpretation: If any of the FSH levels are > 10 mIU/ml or the estradiol is > 70 pg/ml the test is considered abnormal and confirms reduced ovarian reserve.

Genetic testing based on ancestral backgrounds

Ancestral Group	Disease	Screening Test
Caucasian, Native American	Cystic fibrosis	DNA testing
French Canadian, Cajun	Tay-Sachs	Assessment of hexosaminadase enzyme activity or DNA testing
Jewish	Canavan disease	DNA testing
	Cystic fibrosis	DNA testing
	Gaucher disease	DNA testing
	Tay-Sachs	Assessment of hexosaminadase enzyme activity or DNA testing
African, Asian, Cambodia, Caribbean, Central America, India, Indonesia, Laos, Malaysia, Mediterranean, Middle Eastern, Pakistan, Thailand, Turkey, Vietnam	Hemoglobinopathies	CBC, Hgb electrophoresis

American Diabetes Association (ADA) threshold glucose values

Time	Normal	Borderline	Diabetes mellitus
Fasting	< 110 mg/dl	110–125 mg/dl	≥ 126 mg/dl
2-Hour	< 140 mg/dl	140–199 mg/dl	≥ 200 mg/dl

For screening purposes it is recommended to do a fasting blood glucose initially. If the fasting blood glucose is abnormal then a 2-hour glucose tolerance test should be performed. For this test a fasting level is measured, the patient drinks 75 g of glucose and blood is drawn again 2 hours later for a glucose determination

Internet Resources for Reproductive Toxins

Pregnancy and Environmental Hotline
  http://www.thegenesisfund.org/hotline.htm

TOXLINE
  http://toxnet.nlm.nih.gov/cgi-bin/sis/htmlgen?TOXLINE

United States Food and Drug Administration
  http://www.fda.gov/cder/

Physicians Desk Reference
  www.pdr.net

Reprotox
  www.reprotox.org

TERIS & Shepard's Catalog of Teratogenic Agents
  http://depts.washington.edu/~terisweb/

Recurrent Miscarriage Work-up

1. Rule out environmental exposures and lifestyle issues

2. Assessment of ovarian function
   - Menstrual history
   - Cycle 3 – FSH, estradiol, TSH

3. Examination of uterine cavity by one of the following:
   - Hysterosalpingogram
   - Sonohysterogram
   - Hysteroscopy

4. Autoimmune work-up
   - Anticardiolipin antibodies
   - Lupus anticoagulant

5. Chromosomal
   - Karyotypes on both partners

Chromosomal abnormalities in liveborn infants and maternal age*

Maternal Age	Risk for Down's Syndrome	Total Risk for Chromosomal Anomalies†
20	1/1667	1/526
21	1/1667	1/526
22	1/1429	1/500
23	1/1429	1/500
24	1/1250	1/476
25	1/1250	1/476
26	1/1176	1/476
27	1/1111	1/455
28	1/1053	1/435
29	1/1000	1/417
30	1/952	1/385
31	1/909	1/385
32	1/769	1/322
33	1/602	1/286
34	1/485	1/238
35	1/378	1/192
36	1/289	1/156
37	1/224	1/127
38	1/173	1/102
39	1/136	1/83
40	1/106	1/66
41	1/82	1/53
42	1/63	1/42
43	1/49	1/33
44	1/38	1/26
45	1/30	1/21
46	1/23	1/16
47	1/18	1/13
48	1/14	1/10
49	1/11	1/8

* The data presented above were modified from Hook DB, Cross PK, Schreinemachers DM. Chromosomal abnormality rates at amniocentesis and in live-born infants. *J Am Med Assoc* 1983; 249:2034–38, and Hook EB. Rates of chromosomal abnormalities at different maternal ages. *Obstet Gynecol* 1981;58:282–5

† The other chromosomal anomalies that are increased with maternal age in addition to 47,+21 (Down's syndrome) are 47,+18; and 47,+13; 47,XYY (Klinefelter's syndrome); 47,XYY and 47,XXX. The incidence of 47,XXX for women between the ages of 20 and 32 years is not available

BODY MASS INDEX

Height	Normal						Overweight					Obesity										Extreme obesity					
	19	20	21	22	23	24	25	26	27	28	29	30	31	32	33	34	35	36	37	38	39	40	41	42	43	44	45
4'10"	91	96	100	105	110	115	119	124	129	134	138	143	148	153	158	162	167	172	177	181	186	191	196	201	205	210	215
4'11"	94	99	104	109	114	119	124	128	133	138	143	148	153	158	163	168	173	178	183	188	193	196	203	208	212	215	222
5'0"	97	102	107	112	118	123	128	133	138	143	148	153	158	163	169	173	179	184	189	194	199	204	209	215	220	225	230
5'1"	100	106	111	116	122	127	132	137	143	148	153	158	164	169	174	180	185	190	195	201	206	211	217	222	227	232	238
5'2"	104	10	115	120	126	131	136	142	147	153	158	164	169	174	180	185	191	196	202	207	213	218	224	229	235	240	246
5'3"	107	113	118	124	130	135	141	146	152	158	163	169	175	180	185	192	197	203	208	214	220	225	231	237	242	248	254
5'4"	110	116	122	128	134	140	145	151	157	163	169	174	180	186	192	197	204	209	215	221	227	232	238	244	250	256	262
5'5"	114	120	126	132	138	144	150	156	162	168	14	180	186	192	198	204	210	216	222	228	234	240	246	252	258	264	270
5'6"	118	124	130	136	142	148	155	161	167	173	179	186	192	198	204	210	216	223	229	235	241	247	253	260	266	272	278
5'7"	121	127	134	140	146	153	159	166	172	178	185	191	198	204	210	217	223	230	236	242	249	255	261	268	274	280	287
5'8"	125	131	138	144	151	158	164	171	177	184	190	197	203	210	216	223	230	236	243	249	256	262	269	276	282	289	295
5'9"	128	135	142	149	155	162	169	176	182	189	196	203	209	216	223	230	236	243	250	257	263	270	277	284	291	297	304
5'10"	132	139	146	153	160	167	174	181	188	195	202	209	216	222	229	236	243	250	257	264	271	278	285	292	299	306	313
5'11"	136	143	150	157	165	172	179	186	193	200	208	215	222	229	236	243	250	257	265	272	279	286	293	301	308	315	322
6'0"	140	147	154	162	169	177	184	191	199	206	213	221	228	235	242	250	258	265	272	279	287	294	302	309	316	324	331
6'1"	144	151	159	166	174	182	189	197	204	212	219	227	235	242	250	257	265	272	280	288	295	302	310	318	325	333	340
6'2"	148	155	163	171	179	186	194	202	210	218	225	233	241	249	256	264	272	280	287	295	303	311	319	326	334	342	350
6'3"	152	160	168	176	184	192	200	208	216	224	232	240	248	256	264	272	279	287	295	303	311	319	327	335	343	351	359
6'4"	156	164	172	180	189	197	205	213	221	230	238	246	254	263	271	279	287	295	304	312	320	326	339	344	353	361	369

Instructions: Find your patient's height on the far left column, then move to the right to find the weight (lbs) in the corresponding row. Then ascend the column to determine the BMI. For instance, a woman who is 5'6" tall and weighs 229 lbs has a BMI of 37

Medication	Indications	Dosage	Comments
Progesterone	1. Recurrent miscarriages 2. IVF/egg donation treatment 3. Surgical removal of corpus luteum during first trimester 4. See Chapter 8 for detailed description	**Vaginal** – Crinone® 90 mg q.d. – suppositories 100 mg b.i.d. – Prometrium® 200 mg b.i.d. **Oral** – Prometrium 100 mg t.i.d. **Intramuscular** – Progesterone-in-oil available in 10-cc bottles (50 mg/cc); administer 50 mg q.d. (1 cc) by IM injection	1. Natural progesterone medications are *not* associated with an increased risk of birth defects 2. Progesterone can delay the onset of a menstrual period even if the patient is not pregnant 3. Progesterone should be discontinued by 10 weeks of pregnancy

Clomiphene citrate	1. Anovulation
	2. Unexplained infertility
	3. For intrauterine insemination treatment
	4. See Chapter 7 for more detailed description
		50–150 mg cycle days 3–7	1. Common side-effects: hot flushes, visual symptoms, emotional irritability
			2. Multiple pregnancy rate – 10%
			  9% twins
			  1% triplets
			3. Most pregnancies are achieved after 3–4 months of treatment

Metformin	1. Chronic anovulation/polycystic ovarian disease 2. See Chapter 7 for detailed description	1. Metformin is available in 500-mg tablets 2. 500 mg q.d. × 1 week; then 500 mg b.i.d. × 1 week; then 500 mg t.i.d.	1. Check renal and liver studies; fasting glucose 2. Side-effects: gastrointestinal upset including diarrhea 3. See patient every 4–6 weeks. Check pregnancy test if indicated 4. Discontinue metformin with the establishment of pregnancy

Dopaminergic agents
  Parlodel®
  Dostinex®
	1. Hyperprolactinemia
	2. See Chapter 7 for a detailed description
		1. Parlodel – 1.25 mg q.h.s. for 1 week then increase to 2.5 mg q.h.s.
		2. Dostinex – 0.5 mg twice a week
			1. Repeat prolactin level in 2–3 weeks and adjust dose accordingly
			2. Side-effects: gastrointestinal upset, fatigue, dizziness and nasal stuffiness

Dexamethasone	1. Adrenal hyperandrogenism – need to R/O Cushing's disease and adrenal tumor 2. Used in combination with clomiphene citrate 3. See chapter 7 for a detailed description	0.5 mg q.h.s.	1. Check AM cortisol level in 1 month if < 3 µg/dl then the dose should be decreased to 0.25 mg q.h.s. 2. Discontinue when pregnancy is achieved

Success rates for conservative infertility treatment options

Treatment	Success Rate (per cycle) (%)	Multiple Pregnancy Rate (%)
Observation	3–4	1
Non-medicated IUI	4	1
Clomiphene citrate	6	10
Clomiphene citrate–IUI	8–10	10
FSH	10	15–20
FSH–IUI	15–18	20–25

IUI, intrauterine insemination; FSH, follicle stimulating hormone injections

1998 National IVF statistics

Treatment	Live-birth rates by age group (%)				Multiple Pregnancy Rate (%)[†]
	< 35	35–37	38–40	> 40	
IVF (± ICSI)*	32	26	18	8	39[†]
Frozen embryo transfer[‡]	21	19	18	13	N/A
Egg donation[‡]	42	44	40	41	N/A

* Live-birth rates per cycle initiated
[†] percentage of multiple pregnancies includes 28% twin and 11% triplets or more
[‡] live-birth rates per embryo transfer
N/A, not available

References

1. US Department of Health and Human Services. *Fertility, Family planning, and Women's Health*. New data from the 1995 National Survey of Family Growth; Centers for Disease Control and Prevention/National Center for Health Statistics. Series 23, No. 19. US Department of Health and Human Services. May 1997 (*www.cdc.gov/nchs/nsfg.htm*)

2. Levit KR, Lazenby HC, Braden BR, *et al*. National health expenditures, 1995. *Health Care Financing Review* 1996;18:175–214

3. Munne S, Alikani M, Tomkin G, *et al*. Embryo morphology, developmental rates and maternal age are correlated with chromosome abnormalities. *Fertil Steril* 1995;64:382–91

4. Hook EB, Cross PK, Schreinemachers DM. Chromosomal abnormality rates at amniocentesis and in live-born infants. *J Am Med Assoc* 1983;249:2034–8

5. Daling JR, Weiss NS, Metch BJ, *et al*. Primary tubal infertility in relation to the use of an intrauterine device. *N Engl J Med* 1985;312:937–41

6. Doll H, Vessey M, Painter R. Return of fertility in nulliparous women after discontinuation of the intrauterine device: comparison with women discontinuing other methods of contraception. *Br J Obstet Gynaecol* 2001;108:304–14

7. Hatch EE, Bracken MB. Association of delayed conceptions with caffeine consumption. *Am J Epidemiol* 1993;38:1082–92

8. Bolumar F, Olsen J, Rebagliato M, Bisanti L. Caffeine intake and delayed conception: a European multicenter study on infertility and subfecundity. European Study Group on Infertility Subfecundity. *Am J Epidemiol* 1997;145:324–34

9. De Mouzon J, Spira A, Schwartz D. A prospective study of the relation between smoking and fertility. *Int J Epidemiol* 1988;17:378–84

10. Bolumar F, Olsen J, Boldsen J. Smoking reduces fecundity: a European multicenter study on infertility and subfecundity. European Study Group on Infertility Subfecundity. *Am J Epidemiol* 1996;143:578–87

11. *Smoking and Women's Health*. Education Bulletin, Number 240. American College of Obstetricians & Gynecologists, 1997

12. Jensen TK, Hjollund NHI, Henriksen TB, *et al*. Does moderate alcohol consumption affect fertility? Follow up study among couples planning first pregnancy. *Br Med J* 1998;317:505–10

13. Hakim RB, Gray RH, Zacur H. Alcohol and caffeine consumption and decreased fertility. *Fertil Steril* 1998;70:632–7

14. Domar AD, Clapp D, Slawsby EA, *et al*. Impact of group psychological interventions on pregnancy rates in infertile women. *Fertil Steril* 2000;73:805–11

15. Shoup D, Mishell DR Jr, Lacarra M, *et al*. Correlation of endometrial maturation with four methods of estimating day of ovulation. *Obstet Gynecol* 1989;73:88–92

16. Li T-C, Dockery P, Rogers AW, Cooke ID. How precise is histologic dating of endometrium using the standard dating criteria? *Fertil Steril* 1989;51:759–63

17. Batista MC, Cartledge TP, Merino MJ, *et al*. Midluteal phase endometrial biopsy does not accurately predict luteal function. *Fertil Steril* 1993;59:294–300

18. Sharara FI, Scott RT Jr, Seifer DB. The detection of diminished ovarian reserve in infertile women. *Am J Obstet Gynecol* 1998;179:804–12

19. Legro RS, Finegood D, Dunaif A. A fasting glucose to insulin ratio is a useful measure of insulin sensitivity in women with polycystic ovary syndrome. *J Clin Endocrinol Metab* 1998; 83:2694–8

20. Grimes DA. Validity of the postcoital test. *Am J Obstet Gynecol* 1995;172:1327

21. Evers JL, Collins JA, Vandekerckhove P. Surgery or embolisation for varicocele in subfertile men (Cochrane Review). *Cochrane Database Syst Rev* 2001;1:CD000479

22. Stumpf PG, March CM. Febrile morbidity following hystersalpingography: identification of risk factors and recommendations for prophylaxis. *Fertil Steril* 1980;33:487–92

23. Alper MM, Garner PR, Spence JE, Quarrington AM. Pregnancy rates after hysterosalpingography with oil- and water-soluble contrast media. *Obstet Gynecol* 1986;68:6–9

24. Falsetti L, Pasinetti E, Mazzani MD, Gastaldi A. Weight loss and menstrual cycle: clinical and endocrinological evaluation. *Gynecol Endocrinol* 1992;6:49–56

25. Endler GC, Mariona FG, Sokol RJ, *et al.* Anesthesia-related maternal mortality in Michigan, 1972–1984. *Am J Obstet Gynecol* 1988;159:187–93

26. World Health Organization. *Physical Status: the Use and Interpretation of Anthropometry.* Report of a WHO expert committee. WHO Tech. Rep. Ser. 854. Geneva: WHO, 1995

27. Fernandes O, Sabharwal M, Smiley T, *et al.* Moderate to heavy caffeine consumption during pregnancy and relationship to spontaneous abortion and abnormal fetal growth: a meta-analysis. *Reprod Toxicol* 1998;12:435–44

28. Mulinare J, Cordero JF, Erickson JD, Berry RT. Periconceptional use of multivitamins and the occurrence of NTDs. *J Am Med Assoc* 1988;260:3141–5

29. Bower C, Stanley FJ. Dietary folate as a risk factor for NTDs: evidence from a case control study in Western Australia. *Med J Aust* 1989;150:613–19

30. Miles JL, Rhoads GG, Simpson JL, *et al.* The absence of a relationship between the periconceptional use of vitamins and NTDs. *N Engl J Med* 1989;321:430–5

31. Milunsky A, Jick H, Jick SS, *et al.* Multivitamin/folic acid supplementation in early pregnancy reduces the prevalence of NTDs. *J Am Med Assoc* 1989;262:2847–52

32. Shaw GM, Velie EM, Schaffer D. Risk of neural tube defect-affected pregnancies among obese women. *J Am Med Assoc* 1996;275:1093–6

33. MRC Vitamin Study Research Group. Prevention of NTDs: results of the Medical Research Council Vitamin study. *Lancet* 1991;338:131

34. Smithells RW, Nevin NC, Sellers MJ, *et al.* Further experience of vitamin supplementation for the prevention of NTD recurrences. *Lancet* 1983;1:1027

35. Vergel RG, Sanchez LR, Heredero BL, *et al.* Primary prevention of NTDs with folic acid supplementation: Cuban experience. *Prenat Diagn* 1990;10:149

36. Rothman KJ, Moore LL, Singer MR, *et al.* Teratogenicity of high vitamin A intake. *N Engl J Med* 1995;333:1369–73

37. Lammer EJ, Hayes AM, Schunior A, Holmes LB. Unusually high risk for adverse outcomes of pregnancy following fetal isotretinoin exposure. *Am J Hum Genet* 1988;43:A58

38. Ondrizek RR, Chan PJ, Patton WC, King A. An alternative medicine study of herbal effects on the penetration of zona-free hamster oocytes and the integrity of sperm deoxyribonucleic acid. *Fertil Steril* 1999;71:517–22

39. Bayer SR, Turksoy RN, Emmi AM, Reindollar RH. Rubella susceptibility of an infertile population. *Fertil Steril* 1991;56:145–6

40. Reid KC, Grizzard TA, Poland GA. Adult immunizations: recommendations for practice. *Mayo Clin* 1999;74:377–84

41. Rodrigues J, Niederman MS. Pneumonia complicating pregnancy. *Clin Chest Med* 1992; 13:679–91

42. ACOG. *Viral Hepatitis in Pregnancy.* Educational Bulletin, Number 248. ACOG, July 1998

43. Makuc D, Lalich N. Employment characteristics of mothers during pregnancy. *Health United States and Prevention Profile 1983.* National Center for Health Statistics, DHSS Publication No. (PHS) 841232. Washington, DC: US Government Printing Office, December 1983: 25–32

44. Cohen EN, Bellville JW, Brown BW Jr. Anesthesia, pregnancy and miscarriage: a study of operating room nurses and anesthetists. *Anesthesiology* 1971;35:343–7

45. Rowland AS, Baird DD, Weinberg CR, *et al.* Reduced fertility among women employed as dental assistants exposed to high levels of nitrous oxide. *N Engl J Med* 1992;327:993–7

46. Guirguis SS, Pelmear PL, Roy ML, Wong L. Health effects associated with exposure to anesthetic gases in Ontario hospital personnel. *Br J Int Med* 1990;47:490–7

47. John EM, Savitz DA, Shy DM. Spontaneous abortions among cosmetologists. *Epidemiology* 1994;5:147–55

48. Brent RL, Gordon WE, Bennett WR, Beckman DA. Reproductive and teratologic effects of electromagnetic fields. *Reprod Toxicol* 1993;7:535–80

49. Parazzini F, Luchini L, La Vecchia C, Crosignani PG. Video display terminal use during pregnancy and reproductive outcome: a meta-analysis. *J Epidemiol Community Health* 1993; 47:265–8

50. Khattak S, K-Moghtader G, McMartin K, *et al.* Pregnancy outcome following gestational exposure to organic solvents: a prospective controlled study. *J Am Med Assoc* 1999;281: 1106–9

51. Whorton D, Krauss RM, Marshall S, *et al.* Infertility in male pesticide workers. *Lancet* 1977; 2:1259–61

52. Van Voorhis BJ, Barnett M, Sparks AET, *et al.* Prognostic factors for pregnancy following intrauterine insemination and *in vitro* fertilization. *Fertil Steril* 2000;74:S46

53. CDC. *The 1998 Assisted Reproductive Technology Success Rates.* United States Centers for Disease Control (CDC), 1998

54. Whittemore AS, Harris R, Itnyre J, and the Collaborative Ovarian Cancer Group. Characteristics relating to ovarian cancer risk: collaborative analysis of 12 US case–control studies. *Am J Epidemiol* 1992;136:1184–203

55. Rossing MA, Daling JR, Weiss NS, *et al.* Ovarian tumors in a cohort of infertile women. *N Engl J Med* 1994;331:771–6

56. Hughes E, Collins J, Vandekerckhove P. Clomiphene citrate vs placebo or no treatment in unexplained subfertility. *The Cochrane Library, Update Software,* 1999; Issue 4 (Search date not stated; primary source Cochrane menstrual disorders and subfertility groups register of controlled trials)

57. Hughes EG. The effectiveness of ovulation induction and intrauterine insemination in the treatment of persistent infertility: a meta-analysis. *Hum Reprod* 1997;12:1865–72

58. Fujii S, Fukui A, Fukushi Y, *et al.* The effects of clomiphene citrate on normally ovulatory women. *Fertil Steril* 1997;68:997–9

59. Gysler M, March CM, Mishell DR, Bailey EJ. A decade's experience with an individualized clomiphene treatment regimen including its effect on the post-coital test. *Fertil Steril* 1982; 37:161

60. Garcia J, Jones GS, Wentz AC. The use of clomiphene citrate. *Fertil Steril* 1977;28:707

61. Nestler JE, Jakubowicz DJ, Evans WS, Pasquali R. Effects of metformin on spontaneous and clomiphene-induced ovulation in the polycystic ovary syndrome. *N Engl J Med* 1998; 338:1876–80

62. Velazquez EM, Acosta A, Mendoza SG. Menstrual cyclicity after metformin therapy in polycystic ovary syndrome. *Obstet Gynecol* 1997;90:392–5

63. Velazquez EM, Mendoza SG, Hamer, *et al.* Metformin therapy in polycystic ovary syndrome reduces hyperinsulinemia, insulin resistance, hyperandrogenemia, and systolic blood pressure, while facilitating normal menses and pregnancy. *Metabolism* 1994;43:647–54

64. Cuellar FG. Bromocriptine mesylate (Parlodel) in the management of amenorrhea/galactorrhea associated with hyperprolactinemina. *Obstet Gynecol* 1980;55:278

65. McCord ML, Muram D, Buster JE, *et al.* Single serum progesterone as a screen for ectopic pregnancy: exchanging specificity and sensitivity to obtain optimal test performance. *Fertil Steril* 1996;66:513–16

66. Gelder MS, Boots LR, Younger JB. Use of single random serum progesterone value as a diagnostic aid of ectopic pregnancy. *Fertil Steril* 1991;55:497–500

67. McCord ML, Muram D, Buster JE, Arheart KL, Stovall TG, Carson SA. Single serum progesterone as a screen for ectopic pregnancy: exchanging specificity and sensitivity to obtain optimal test performance. *Fertil Steril* 1996;66:513–16

68. Filicori M, Butler JP, Crowley WF. Neuroendocrine regulation of the corpus luteum in the human: evidence for pulsatile progesterone secretion. *J Clin Invest* 1984;73:1638

69. Schmidt KLT, Ziebe S, Popovic B, *et al.* Progesterone supplementation during early gestation after *in vitro* fertilization has no effect on the delivery rate. *Fertil Steril* 2001;75:337–41

70. Miles RA, Paulson RJ, Lobo RA, *et al*. Pharmacokinetics and endometrial tissue levels of progesterone after administration by intramuscular and vaginal routes; a comparative study. *Fertil Steril* 1994;62:485–90

71. Lipscomb GH, Stovall TG, Ling FW. Primary care: nonsurgical treatment of ectopic pregnancy. *N Engl J Med* 2000;343:1325–9

72. Kadar N, Caldwell BV, Romero R. A method of screening for ectopic pregnancy and its indications. *Obstet Gynecol* 1981;58:162–6

73. Pittaway DE, Reish RL, Wentz AC. Doubling times of human chorionic gonadotropin increase in early viable intrauterine pregnancies. *Am J Obstet Gynecol* 1985;152:299–302

74. Shalev E, Peleg D, Tsabari A, *et al*. Spontaneous resolution of ectopic tubal pregnancy: natural history. *Fertil Steril* 1995;63:15–19

75. Korhonen J, Stenman UH, Ylostalo P. Serum human chorionic gonadotropin dynamics during spontaneous resolution of ectopic pregnancy. *Fertil Steril* 1994;61:632–6

76. Corsan GH, Karacan M, Qasim S, *et al*. Identification of hormonal parameters for successful systemic single-dose methotrexate therapy in ectopic pregnancy. *Hum Reprod* 1995;10:2719–22

77. Henry MA, Gentry WL. Single injection of Methotrexate for treatment of ectopic pregnancies. *Am J Obstet Gynecol* 1994;171:1584–7

78. Stika CS, Anderson L, Frederiksen MC. Single-dose methotrexate for the treatment of ectopic pregnancy: Northwester Memorial Hospital three-year experience. *Am J Obstet Gynecol* 1996;174:1840–6

79. Stovall TG, Ling FW. Single dose Methotrexate: an expanded clinical trial. *Am J Obstet Gynecol* 1993;168:1759–65

80. Lipscomb GH, McCord ML, Stovall TG, *et al*. Predictors of success of methotrexate treatment in women with tubal ectopic pregnancies. *N Engl J Med* 1999;341:1974–8

Index